T0294389

PAIN MEDICINE
A CASE-BASED LEARNING SERIES

The Chest Wall and Abdomen

PAIN MEDICINE
A CASE-BASED LEARNING SERIES

The Chest Wall and Abdomen

STEVEN D. WALDMAN, MD, JD

ELSEVIER

Elsevier
1600 John F. Kennedy Blvd.
Ste 1800
Philadelphia, PA 19103-2899

PAIN MEDICINE: A CASE-BASED LEARNING SERIES   ISBN: 978-0-323-84688-2
THE CHEST WALL AND ABDOMEN

Notice

Practitioners and researchers must always rely on their own experience and knowledge in evaluating and using any information, methods, compounds or experiments described herein. Because of rapid advances in the medical sciences, in particular, independent verification of diagnoses and drug dosages should be made. To the fullest extent of the law, no responsibility is assumed by Elsevier, authors, editors or contributors for any injury and/or damage to persons or property as a matter of products liability, negligence or otherwise, or from any use or operation of any methods, products, instructions, or ideas contained in the material herein.

Executive Content Strategist: Michael Houston
Content Development Specialist: Jeannine Carrado/Laura Klein
Director, Content Development: Ellen Wurm-Cutter
Publishing Services Manager: Shereen Jameel
Senior Project Manager: Karthikeyan Murthy
Design Direction: Amy Buxton

Printed in India.

Last digit is the print number: 9 8 7 6 5 4 3 2 1

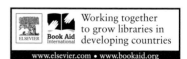

"When you go after honey with a balloon, the great thing is to not let the bees know you're coming."

WINNIE THE POOH

It's Harder Than It Looks
MAKING THE CASE FOR CASE-BASED LEARNING

For sake of full disclosure, I was one of those guys. You know, the ones who wax poetic about how hard it is to teach our students how to do procedures. Let me tell you, teaching folks how to do epidurals on women in labor certainly takes its toll on the coronary arteries. It's true, I am amazing ... I am great ... I have nerves of steel. Yes, I could go on like this for hours ... but you have heard it all before. But, it's again that time of year when our new students sit eagerly before us, full of hopes and dreams ... and that harsh reality comes slamming home ... it is a lot harder to teach beginning medical students "doctoring" than it looks.

A few years ago, I was asked to teach first-year medical and physician assistant students how to take a history and perform a basic physical exam. In my mind, I thought, "This should be easy ... no big deal." I won't have to do much more than show up. After all, I was the guy who wrote that amazing book on physical diagnosis. After all, I had been teaching medical students, residents, and fellows how to do highly technical (and dangerous, I might add) interventional pain management procedures since right after the Civil War. Seriously, it was no big deal ... I could do it in my sleep ... with one arm tied behind my back ... blah ... blah ... blah.

For those of you who have had the privilege of teaching "doctoring," you already know what I am going to say next. *It's harder than it looks!* Let me repeat this to disabuse any of you who, like me, didn't get it the first time. *It is harder than it looks!* I only had to meet with my first-year medical and physician assistant students a couple of times to get it through my thick skull: **It really is harder than it looks**. In case you are wondering, the reason that our students look back at us with those blank, confused, bored, and ultimately dismissive looks is simple: They lack context. That's right, they lack the context to understand what we are talking about.

It's really that simple ... or hard ... depending on your point of view or stubbornness, as the case may be. To understand why context is king, you have to look only as far as something as basic as the Review of Systems. The Review of Systems is about as basic as it gets, yet why is it so perplexing to our students? Context. I guess it should come as no surprise to anyone that the student is completely lost when you talk about ... let's say ... the "constitutional" portion of the Review of Systems, without the context of what a specific constitutional finding, say a fever or chills, might mean to a patient who is suffering from the acute onset of headaches. If you tell the student that you need to ask about fever, chills, and the other "constitutional" stuff and you take it no further, you might as well be talking about the

International Space Station. Just save your breath; it makes absolutely no sense to your students. Yes, they want to please, so they will memorize the elements of the Review of Systems, but that is about as far as it goes. On the other hand, if you present the case of Jannette Patton, a 28-year-old first-year medical resident with a fever and headache, you can see the lights start to come on. By the way, this is what Jannette looks like, and as you can see, Jannette is sicker than a dog. This, at its most basic level, is what *Case-Based Learning* is all about.

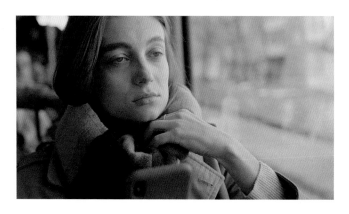

I would like to tell you that, smart guy that I am, I immediately saw the light and became a convert to *Case-Based Learning*. But truth be told, it was COVID-19 that really got me thinking about *Case-Based Learning*. Before the COVID-19 pandemic, I could just drag the students down to the med/surg wards and walk into a patient room and riff. Everyone was a winner. For the most part, the patients loved to play along and thought it was cool. The patient and the bedside was all I needed to provide the context that was necessary to illustrate what I was trying to teach—the "why headache and fever don't mix" kind of stuff. Had COVID-19 not rudely disrupted my ability to teach at the bedside, I suspect that you would not be reading this *Preface*, as I would not have had to write it. Within a very few days after the COVID-19 pandemic hit, my days of bedside teaching disappeared, but my students still needed context. This got me focused on how to provide the context they needed. The answer was, of course, *Case-Based Learning*. What started as a desire to provide context . . . because it really was **harder than it looked** . . . led me to begin work on this eight-volume *Case-Based Learning* textbook series. What you will find within these volumes are a bunch of fun, real-life cases that help make each patient come alive for the student. These cases provide the contextual teaching points that make it easy for the teacher to explain why, when Jannette's chief complaint is, *"My head is killing me and I've got a fever,"* it is a big deal.

Have fun!

Steven D. Waldman, MD, JD
Spring 2021

ACKNOWLEDGMENTS

A very special thanks to my editors, Michael Houston, PhD, Jeannine Carrado, and Karthikeyan Murthy, for all their hard work and perseverance in the face of disaster. Great editors such as Michael, Jeannine, and Karthikeyan make their authors look great, for they not only understand how to bring the Three Cs of great writing. . .Clarity + Consistency + Conciseness. . .to the author's work, but unlike me, they can actually punctuate and spell!

Steven D. Waldman, MD, JD

P.S. . . .Sorry for all the ellipses, guys!

CONTENTS

13 **Brian Nguyen** A 23-Year-Old With Severe Testicular Pain and
Hematuria   182

14 **Vivian Zhao** A 32-Year-Old Female With Right Lower Quadrant
Pain   200

15 **Mai Huang** A 64-Year-Old Waitress With Left-Sided Abdominal
Pain and Fever   216

Index   231

Thomas Wang

A 28-Year-Old Stockbroker With Severe Anterior Chest Pain

LEARNING OBJECTIVES

- Learn the common causes of chest wall pain.
- Develop an understanding of the unique anatomy of the chest wall.
- Develop an understanding of the causes of costosternal joint pain.
- Develop an understanding of joint injury.
- Learn the clinical presentation of costosternal syndrome.
- Learn how to use physical examination to identify pathology of the costosternal joint.
- Develop an understanding of the treatment options for costosternal joint pain.

Thomas Wang

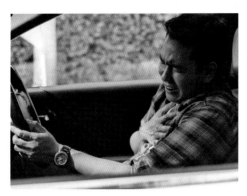

Thomas Wang is a 28-year-old stockbroker with the chief complaint of, "My chest is killing me." Thomas stated that about 1 week ago, he was involved in a motor vehicle accident when driving home from a party. "A dog ran out of nowhere and startled me, and the next thing I remember is waking up after crashing into a tree. The good news is I didn't hit the dog; the bad news is I got a DUI. I had a couple of glasses of wine with my friends, but thought I was okay to drive home." I asked if he was wearing his seatbelt and he gave me an "are you kidding me?" look as he answered that he always wears his seatbelt. "Doctor, I don't know whether it was the seatbelt or the airbag that got my chest, but it hurts whenever I take a deep breath or reach for anything. I had to buy some go-cups because I can't get my coffee mugs out of the cabinet! I thought it would get better, but it really hasn't." I responded, "I'm happy to hear you were wearing your seatbelt. So, did you hit your head?" He said he didn't think so, that he thought he just fell asleep after he hit the tree. They took him to the emergency room, and the scan of his head didn't show anything. "Doctor, I really screwed up here. I hope I don't lose my license for this little stunt. My blood alcohol was off the charts! I can't figure it out; it was only a couple of glasses of wine. I really bunged up my chest. They said nothing was broken, so why does it hurt so much?"

I asked Thomas if he had anything like this happen before. He shook his head and responded, "Never. I never drink and drive. I usually take an Uber, but they were on price surge, and that is just a rip-off. I was sure I was good to drive." "What I meant, Thomas, was have you ever passed out or lost consciousness?" "No," he responded. "That has never happened. I am very careful with the distracted driving and all—you know what I mean? What worries me is that my chest just isn't getting better, and it is making it really hard to sit at a computer monitor all day. It feels like something is broken in the front of my chest. I am even having a hard time reaching up to wash my hair and to shave."

I asked Thomas about any previous problems with alcohol, passing out, DUIs, or forgetting where he was, and he shook his head no. "Doc, I was never much of a drinker, just a couple glasses of wine with dinner. I really enjoy the California reds." I asked Thomas what he tried to relieve his chest pain, and he said that he had tried some Advil and Tylenol, but they didn't do much. He went on to say that a heating pad seemed to help a little bit. I asked Thomas what made his pain worse, and he said, "Any time I use my arms to reach for anything or take a deep breath. I hate it when I have to cough or sneeze because that really hurts." Thomas went on to say that when he reached up, he felt pain in the front of his chest around his breast bone. I asked how he was sleeping, and he shook his head and said, "Doc, I'll bet this pain wakes me up 100 times a night. I usually sleep on my left side, but since I had the wreck I can't do that, so I try to sleep on my right side. Every time I roll over to my left side, the pain wakes me up."

I asked Thomas to point with one finger to show me where it hurt the most. He pointed to each side of his sternum and said, "Doc, it's right here where something is wrong. It feels like something is broken. I keep thinking there should be a bruise or something, but it's down deep." I asked if he had any fever or chills, and he shook his head no.

On physical examination, Thomas was afebrile. His respirations were 16 and his pulse was 68 and regular. His blood pressure was 112/70. His head, eyes, ears, nose, throat (HEENT) exam was normal, with no scleral icterus. His cardio-pulmonary examination was unremarkable. His thyroid was normal. His abdominal examination revealed no abnormal mass or organomegaly; specifi-cally, I was unable to detect any hepatomegaly. There was no costovertebral angle (CVA) tenderness or peripheral edema. His low back examination was unremarkable. Visual inspection of the chest wall was unremarkable; specifi-cally, there was no obvious bony deformity or infection. I noted that Thomas was splinting his shoulders a little forward to avoid moving his chest wall. Palpation of the costosternal joints exacerbated Thomas's pain (Fig. 1.1). I did not appreciate any obvious separation of the costosternal joint. I performed the shoulder retraction test for costosternal syndrome, which was positive bilater-ally (Fig. 1.2). Examination of the joints of the hands and other major joints revealed no evidence of inflammatory arthritis. A careful neurologic examina-tion of the upper extremities revealed no evidence of peripheral or entrapment neuropathy, and the deep tendon reflexes were normal. Thomas's mental status examination was normal.

Key Clinical Points—What's Important and What's Not
THE HISTORY

- A history of acute trauma to the chest wall from an airbag and seatbelt
- A history of motor vehicle accident
- History of driving while intoxicated
- History of daily alcohol intake
- No history of previous significant chest wall pain
- No fever or chills

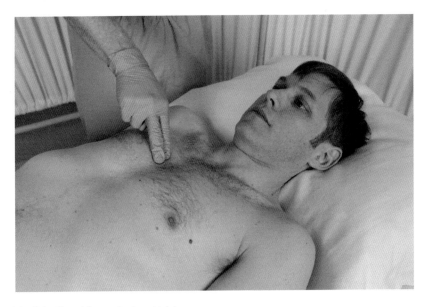

Fig. 1.1 Palpation of the costosternal joint.

- Exacerbation of pain with deep inspiration and elevation of the upper extremities
- Sleep disturbance

THE PHYSICAL EXAMINATION

- Patient is afebrile
- Palpation of costosternal joints reveals tenderness bilaterally (see Fig. 1.1)
- No evidence of infection
- Shoulder retraction test for costosternal syndrome positive bilaterally (see Fig. 1.2)

OTHER FINDINGS OF NOTE

- Normal HEENT examination
- Normal cardiovascular examination
- Normal pulmonary examination
- Normal abdominal examination
- No peripheral edema
- Normal upper extremity neurologic examination, motor and sensory examination
- Examination of other joints normal

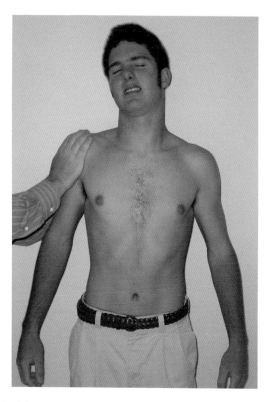

Fig. 1.2 To elicit a shoulder retraction test in patients who are suspected of suffering from costosternal syndrome, the patient is placed in the standing position with the shoulders in neutral position, facing the examiner. The patient is then asked to retract the shoulder vigorously. The shoulder retraction test is considered positive if the retraction maneuver reproduces the patient's anterior chest wall pain. (From Waldman S. *Physical Diagnosis of Pain: An Atlas of Signs and Symptoms*. ed. 4. Philadelphia: Elsevier; 2021 [Fig. 143-1].)

What Tests Would You Like to Order?

The following tests were ordered:
- Plain radiographs of the chest wall
- Complete blood count
- Comprehensive chemistry panel, including liver enzymes

TEST RESULTS

The plain radiographs of the sternum and costosternal joints revealed no fractures or dislocations.

The complete blood count revealed no megaloblastic anemia.

The comprehensive chemistry panel was within normal limits with no elevation of liver enzymes.

Clinical Correlation—Putting it all Together

What is the diagnosis?
- Costosternal syndrome secondary to acute traumatic injury

The Science Behind the Diagnosis

ANATOMY OF THE COSTOSTERNAL JOINTS

The cartilage of the true ribs articulates with the sternum via the costosternal joints (Fig. 1.3). The cartilage of the first rib articulates directly with the manubrium of the sternum and is a synarthrodial joint that allows a limited gliding movement. The cartilage of the second through sixth ribs articulates with the body of the sternum via true arthrodial joints. These joints are surrounded by a thin articular capsule. The costosternal joints are strengthened by ligaments but

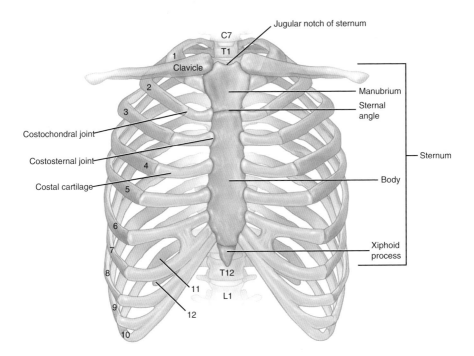

Fig. 1.3 The anatomy of the chest wall. (From Waldman S. *Atlas of Pain Management Injection Techniques*. ed. 4. St. Louis: Elsevier; 2017 [Fig. 99-3].)

can be subluxed or dislocated by blunt trauma to the anterior chest. Posterior to the costosternal joint are the structures of the mediastinum. These structures are susceptible to needle-induced trauma if the needle is placed too deeply. The pleural space may be entered if the needle is placed too deeply and laterally, and pneumothorax may result.

CLINICAL SYNDROME

Many patients with noncardiogenic chest pain suffer from costosternal joint pain. Most commonly, the costosternal joints become painful in response to inflammation as a result of overuse or misuse, or in response to trauma secondary to acceleration-deceleration injuries or blunt trauma to the chest wall (Fig. 1.4). With severe trauma, the joints may subluxate or dislocate. The costosternal joints are

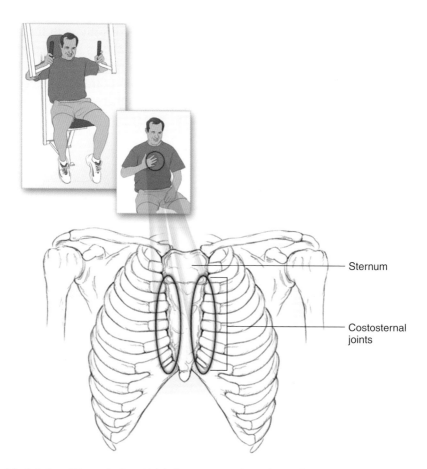

Sternum

Costosternal joints

Fig. 1.4   Irritation of the costosternal joints from overuse of exercise equipment can cause costosternal syndrome. (From Waldman S. *Atlas of Common Pain Syndromes*. ed. 4. Philadelphia: Elsevier; 2019 [Fig. 61-1].)

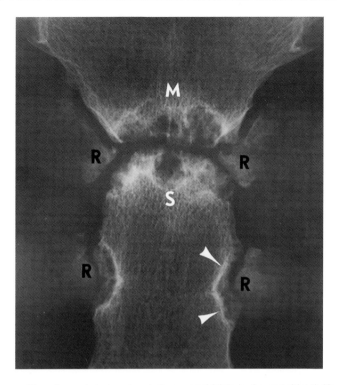

Fig. 1.5 Abnormalities of manubriosternal and sternocostal joints in rheumatoid arthritis. Radiograph of a sternum from a cadaver with rheumatoid arthritis shows large erosions of the articular surface of both the manubrium *(M)* and the body of the sternum *(S)*. Subtle irregularities of the second and third sternocostal joints are evident, most prominently in the sternal facet of the left third sternocostal joint *(arrowheads)*. R, Ossified costal cartilage. (From Resnick D. *Diagnosis of Bone and Joint Disorders*. ed. 4. Philadelphia: Saunders; 2002:854.)

susceptible to the development of osteoarthritis, rheumatoid arthritis, ankylosing spondylitis, Reiter syndrome, and psoriatic arthritis. The joints are also subject to invasion by tumor from primary malignant tumors, including thymoma, or from metastatic disease.

SIGNS AND SYMPTOMS

Physical examination reveals that the patient vigorously attempts to splint the joints by keeping the shoulders stiffly in a neutral position. Pain is reproduced with active protraction or retraction of the shoulder, deep inspiration, full elevation of the arm, and palpation of the costosternal joints (see Fig. 1.1). Patients with painful costosternal joints will exhibit a positive costosternal retraction test (see Fig. 1.2). Shrugging of the shoulder may also reproduce the pain. Coughing may be difficult, leading to inadequate pulmonary toilet in patients who have

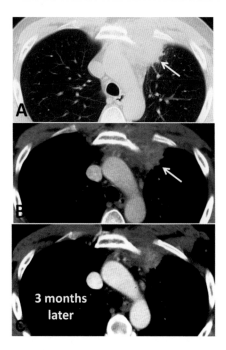

Fig. 1.6 Computed tomography (CT) scan of a patient with anterior chest wall pain. CT scanning of anterior upper mediastinal mass after iodinated contrast administration. Lung window (A). Mediastinum window (B) shows inhomogeneous contrast enhancement of the mass. Enhanced multidetector CT follow-up after 3 months (C) shows decrease in volume of mediastinal mass. (From De Filippo M, Albini A, Castaldi V, et al. MRI findings of Tietze's syndrome mimicking mediastinal malignancy on MDCT. *Eur J Radiol Extra*. 2008;65(1):33—35 [Fig. 1]. ISSN 1571-4675, https://doi.org/10.1016/j.ejrex.2007.10.006, http://www.sciencedirect.com/science/article/pii/S1571467507000892.)

sustained trauma to the anterior chest wall. The costosternal joints and adjacent intercostal muscles may be tender to palpation. The patient may also complain of a clicking sensation with joint movement.

TESTING

Plain radiographs are indicated for all patients who present with pain that is thought to be emanating from the costosternal joints to rule out occult bony disorders, including tumor (Fig. 1.5). If trauma is present, radionuclide bone scanning may be useful to exclude occult fractures of the ribs or sternum. Based on the patient's clinical presentation, additional testing may be indicated, including a complete blood count, prostate-specific antigen level, erythrocyte sedimentation rate, and antinuclear antibody testing. Laboratory evaluation for collagen vascular disease is indicated in patients suffering from costosternal joint pain if other joints are involved. Computed tomography

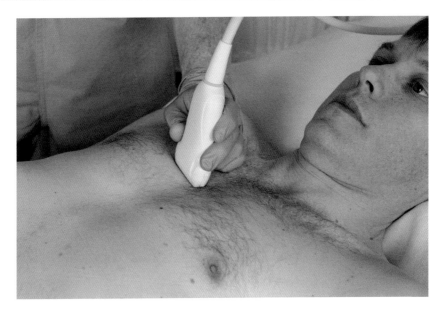

Fig. 1.7 Proper placement of the high-frequency linear ultrasound probe for ultrasound evaluation of the costosternal joint.

(CT) scanning, magnetic resonance imaging (MRI), and ultrasound imaging of the joints are indicated if joint instability or occult mass is suspected, or to elucidate the cause of the pain further (Figs. 1.6, 1.7, and 1.8). Injection of the costosternal joint can serve as both a diagnostic and a therapeutic maneuver (Figs. 1.9 and 1.10).

DIFFERENTIAL DIAGNOSIS

As mentioned, the pain of costosternal syndrome is often mistaken for pain of cardiac origin, and it leads to visits to the emergency department and unnecessary cardiac workups. If trauma has occurred, costosternal syndrome may coexist with fractured ribs or fractures of the sternum itself, which can be missed on plain radiographs and may require CT or radionuclide bone scanning for proper identification (Fig. 1.11). Tietze syndrome, which is painful enlargement of the upper costochondral cartilage associated with viral infection, may be confused with costosternal syndrome (Box 1.1).

Neuropathic pain involving the chest wall may also be confused or coexist with costosternal syndrome. Examples of such neuropathic pain syndromes include diabetic polyneuropathies and acute herpes zoster involving the thoracic nerves. Diseases of the structures of the mediastinum and chest wall may

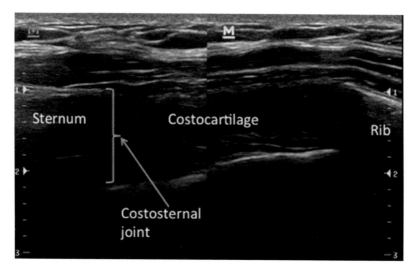

Fig. 1.8   Transverse ultrasound image of the costosternal joint.

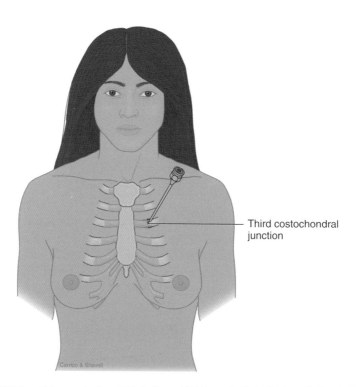

Fig. 1.9   Injection of the costosternal joint. (From Waldman S. *Pain Review*. 2nd. ed. Philadelphia: Elsevier; 2017:9780323448895 [Fig. 286-1].)

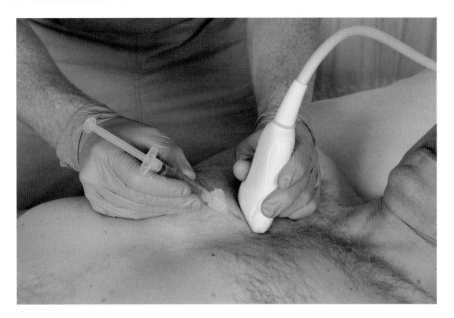

Fig. 1.10   Proper needle placement for ultrasound-guided injection of the costosternal joint.

mimic the pain of costosternal syndrome and may be difficult to diagnose (Fig. 1.12). Pathologic processes that inflame the pleura, such as pulmonary embolus, infection, and Bornholm disease, may also confuse the diagnosis and complicate treatment.

TREATMENT

Initial treatment of the pain and functional disability associated with costosternal syndrome includes a combination of nonsteroidal antiinflammatory drugs (NSAIDs) or cyclooxygenase-2 inhibitors. The local application of heat and cold may also be beneficial. Use of an elastic rib belt may provide symptomatic relief and protect the costosternal joints from additional trauma. For patients who do not respond to these treatment modalities, injection with local anesthetic and steroid is a reasonable next step (see Figs. 1.9 and 1.10). Physical modalities, including local heat and gentle range-of-motion exercises, should be introduced several days after the patient undergoes injection for costosternal joint pain. Vigorous exercises should be avoided because they will exacerbate the patient's symptoms. Simple analgesics and NSAIDs may be used concurrently with this injection technique.

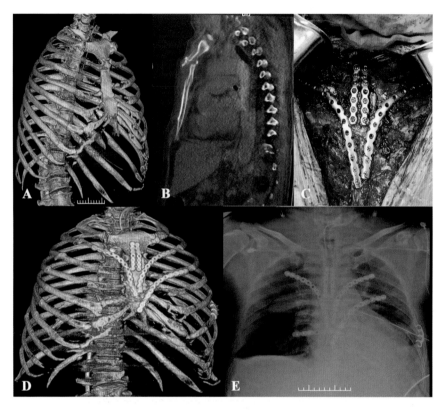

Fig. 1.11 Crush injury of the chest with massive chest wall trauma. (A) Computed tomographic (CT) three-dimensional reconstruction image of the chest wall on admission. (B) CT image of the sternum. (C) Surgical procedure: fixation of sternal and multiple costal cartilage fractures. (D) CT three-dimensional reconstruction image of the chest wall after operation. (E) Chest film obtained 4 days after operation. (From Gao E, Li Y, Zhao T, et al. Simultaneous surgical treatment of sternum and costal cartilage fractures. *Ann Thorac Surg.* 2019;107(2):e119—e120 [Fig. 1]. ISSN 0003-4975, https://doi.org/10.1016/j.athoracsur.2018.06.044, http://www.sciencedirect.com/science/article/pii/S0003497518310488.)

BOX 1.1 ■ Musculoskeletal Chest Wall Pain

Pain Arising From the Joints of the Chest Wall

- Strain of the costosternal joint
- Manubriosternal arthritis
- Tietze syndrome
- Costochondritis
- Xiphodynia
- Costovertebral joint disorders
- Septic arthritis

Pain Arising From the Ribs

- Rib trauma

(Continued)

- Rib fracture
- Primary and metastatic neoplasm of the rib infection
- Slipping rib syndrome

Pain Arising From the Soft Tissues

- Myositis
- Muscle strain
- Fibromyalgia
- Myofascial pain

Miscellaneous Sources of Pain

- Precordial catch syndrome
- Acute herpes zoster
- Zoster sine herpete
- Somatiform disorders

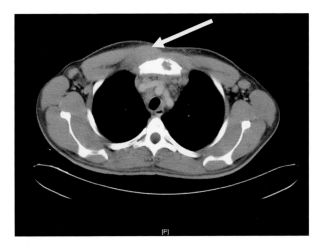

Fig. 1.12 Computed tomography scan of a patient complaining of right costosternal pain revealing a right chest wall mass at the level of the second rib *(arrow)*. (From Rich BS, McEvoy MP, Honeyman JN, et al. Hodgkin lymphoma presenting with chest wall involvement: a case series. *J Pediatr Surg.* 2011;46(9):1835–1837 [Fig. 2]. ISSN 0022-3468, https://doi.org/10.1016/j.jpedsurg.2011.05.015, http://www.sciencedirect.com/science/article/pii/S0022346811004428.)

COMPLICATIONS AND PITFALLS

Because many pathologic processes can mimic the pain of costosternal syndrome, the clinician must carefully rule out underlying cardiac disease and diseases of the lung and structures of the mediastinum. Failure to do so could lead to disastrous results. The major complication of the injection technique is pneumothorax if the needle is placed too laterally or deeply and invades the pleural space. Infection, although rare, can occur if strict aseptic technique is not followed. Trauma to the contents of the mediastinum is also a possibility. The risk of this complication can be greatly decreased with the use of ultrasound guidance for needle placement.

HIGH-YIELD TAKEAWAYS

- The patient is afebrile, making an acute infectious etiology (e.g., septic arthritis) unlikely.
- The patient's symptomatology is the result of acute trauma, and physical examination and testing should focus on the identification of other pathologic processes that may mimic the clinical presentation of costosternal syndrome.
- The patient's pain is localized to the costosternal joints.
- The patient's symptoms involve only the costovertebral joints, which is more suggestive of a local process than a systemic polyarthropathy.
- Sleep disturbance is common and must be addressed concurrently with the patient's pain symptomatology.
- Plain radiographs will provide high-yield information regarding the bony contents of the costovertebral joints, but CT scanning, ultrasound imaging, and MRI will be more useful in identifying soft tissue pathology.

Suggested Readings

Ayloo A, Cvengros T, Marella S. Evaluation and treatment of musculoskeletal chest pain. *Prim Care*. 2013;40(4):863–887.

Hillen TJ, Wessell DE. Multidetector CT scan in the evaluation of chest pain of nontraumatic musculoskeletal origin. *Thorac Surg Clin*. 2010;20(1):167–173.

Lu CH, Hsieh SC, Li KJ. Tophi in anterior chest wall. *Joint Bone Spine*. 2014;81(4):366.

Stochkendahl MJ, Christensen HW. Chest pain in focal musculoskeletal disorders. *Med Clin North Am*. 2010;94(2):259–273.

Waldman SD. Arthritis and other abnormalities of the costosternal joint. In: *Waldman's Comprehensive Atlas of Diagnostic Ultrasound of Painful Conditions*. ed. 2. Philadelphia: Wolters Kluwer; 2016:513–518.

Waldman SD. Costosternal joint injection. In: *Pain Review*. ed. 2. Philadelphia: Elsevier; 2017:462–463.

Waldman SD. Costosternal joint injection technique for Tietze syndrome. In: *Atlas of Pain Management Injection Techniques*. ed. 4. Philadelphia: Elsevier; 2017:349–351.

Waldman SD. Ultrasound-guided injection technique for costosternal joint pain. In: *Waldman's Comprehensive Atlas of Ultrasound Guided Pain Management Injection Techniques*. ed. 2. Philadelphia: Wolters Kluwer; 2020:591–594.

Pete Wilder

A 23-Year-Old Printer With Persistent Chest Wall Pain Following CPR

- Learn the common causes of chest wall pain.
- Develop an understanding of the anatomy of the manubriosternal joint.
- Develop an understanding of the unique clinical presentation of manubriosternal joint pain.
- Develop an understanding of the differential diagnosis of chest wall pain.
- Learn how to use physical examination to identify the manubriosternal joint as the source of chest wall pain.
- Develop an understanding of the treatment options for manubriosternal joint pain.

Pete Wilder

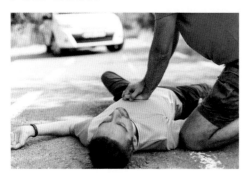

Pete Wilder is a 23-year-old printer with the chief complaint of, "Every time I take a deep breath, it feels like somebody is stabbing me in the chest with a knife." Pete stated that he stopped to help a woman in a mini-van full of kids who was trying to change a tire. The next thing he knew, he woke up in the intensive care unit of the university medical center. "Doctor, I guess I was trying to lift the spare up onto the wheel when a guy in a pickup truck came over the hill and knocked me into next week. A bystander decided I didn't have a pulse and started CPR. He must have really pumped the hell out of my chest because now my breastbone clicks with every breath. The ICU doctor said I had a dislocation or something."

"Doctor, I consider myself a pretty tough guy—you know, I joined the Marines right out of high school—but any time I cough or sneeze, the pain is so bad I just want to scream. It really, really hurts."

I asked Pete if he had experienced any pain or had any previous injury or surgery of the chest wall before all this started, and he shook his head no and replied, "I am as healthy as a horse. I guess no good deed goes unpunished. I guess I am lucky that I didn't get killed trying to help that lady. I really don't remember getting hit by the car or getting my chest pounded on. I guess that's a good thing—or not!?" I asked, "How is your sleep?" Pete replied, "I'm sleeping in my recliner because it keeps me from rolling over, which really hurts. Even then, I bet the pain wakes me up 50 times a night. My boss has been pretty nice about the whole thing, but printing is a pretty physical activity."

I asked Pete to show me the location of the pain, and he pointed to the center of his sternum. "It hurts right here. It's right here, and this is where the clicking comes from, right here." I asked Pete about any fever, chills, or other constitutional symptoms such as weight loss or night sweats, and he shook his head no. He denied any other musculoskeletal or systemic symptoms.

On physical examination, Pete was afebrile. His respirations were 18, his pulse was 74 and regular, and his blood pressure was 124/76. Pete's head, eyes, ears, nose, throat (HEENT) exam was normal, as was his thyroid exam. Auscultation of his carotids revealed no bruits, and the pulses in all four extremities were normal. He had a regular rhythm without abnormal beats. His cardiac exam was otherwise unremarkable. His abdominal examination revealed no abnormal mass or organomegaly. There was no peripheral edema. His low back examination was unremarkable, although flexion of the lumbar

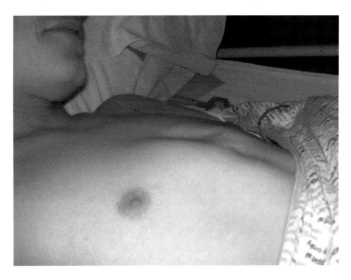

Fig. 2.1 Photograph showing an obvious step-off in the manubriosternal joint following dislocation. (From Lyons I, Saha S, Arulampalam T. Manubriosternal joint dislocation: an unusual risk of trampolining. *J Emerg Med*. 2010;39:596–598.)

spine caused some pain in the right buttocks. There was no costovertebral angle (CVA) tenderness. Visual inspection of Pete's anterior chest wall was unremarkable. There was no evidence of ecchymosis or obvious swelling. Pressure on the sternum caused Pete to cry out in pain. There was an obvious bony deformity with a clearly defined step-off of the manubriosternal joint, suggestive of a manubriosternal dislocation (Fig. 2.1). Pete said, "I've had about all the fun with the poking around that I can stand. Are you about done?" "Sorry, Pete, I just want to figure out what we need to do to get you better. We are about done here." Careful neurologic examinations of both the upper and lower extremities were normal. Deep tendon reflexes were physiologic throughout. "I am pretty sure I know what is causing the pain, and we should be able to get you better."

Key Clinical Points—What's Important and What's Not

THE HISTORY

- History of severe midsternal pain after receiving CPR
- Pain made worse with pressure on the manubriosternal joint
- No history of previous chest or chest wall pain
- No fever or chills
- Significant sleep disturbance

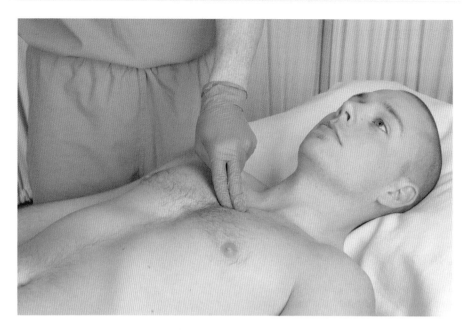

Fig. 2.2 Palpation of the manubriosternal joint.

THE PHYSICAL EXAMINATION

- Patient is afebrile
- Pain on pressure to the midsternum (Fig. 2.2)
- No obvious ecchymosis or swelling
- No obvious deformity of the sternum or manubriosternal joint

OTHER FINDINGS OF NOTE

- Normal HEENT examination
- Normal cardiovascular examination
- Normal pulmonary examination
- Normal abdominal examination
- No peripheral edema

What Tests Would You Like to Order?

The following tests were ordered:
- X-ray of the sternum
- Ultrasound of the manubriosternal joint

TEST RESULTS

X-ray of the sternum was unremarkable with no fracture or bony abnormality. Ultrasound of the manubriosternal joint was reported as normal (Fig. 2.3).

 ## Clinical Correlation—Putting It All Together

What is the diagnosis?
- Manubriosternal joint pain

The Science Behind the Diagnosis

ANATOMY

The manubrium articulates with the body of the sternum via the manubriosternal joint. The joint articulates at an angle called the angle of Louis, which allows for easy identification (Fig. 2.4). The joint is a fibrocartilaginous joint or synchondrosis, which lacks a true joint cavity. The manubriosternal joint allows protraction and retraction of the thorax. Above, the manubrium articulates with the sternal end of the clavicle and the cartilage of the first rib. Below, the body of the sternum articulates with the xiphoid process. Posterior to the manubriosternal joint are the structures of the mediastinum. These structures are susceptible to needle-induced trauma if the needle is placed too deeply. The pleural space may be entered if the needle is placed too deeply and laterally, and pneumothorax may result.

CLINICAL SYNDROME

Pain originating from the manubriosternal joint can mimic pain of cardiac origin. The manubriosternal joint is susceptible to the development of osteoarthritis, rheumatoid arthritis, ankylosing spondylitis, Reiter syndrome, and psoriatic arthritis. The joint can also be traumatized during acceleration-deceleration injuries and blunt trauma to the chest (Figs. 2.5 and 2.6). With severe trauma, the joint may subluxate or dislocate, with the dislocation classified on the basis of the position of the sternum relative to the manubrium (Fig. 2.7). Overuse or misuse can result in acute inflammation of the manubriosternal joint, which can be quite debilitating. The joint is also subject to invasion by tumor from primary malignant tumors, including thymoma, or from metastatic disease. Rarely, septic arthritis of the manubriosternal joint can occur (Fig. 2.8).

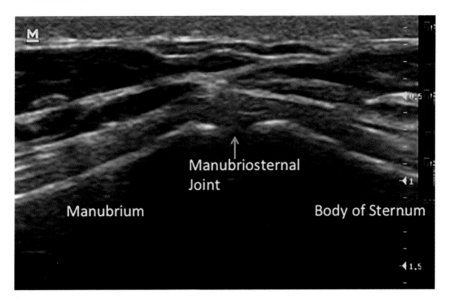

Fig. 2.3   Longitudinal ultrasound image of the manubriosternal joint.

SIGNS AND SYMPTOMS

Physical examination reveals that the patient vigorously attempts to splint the joint by keeping the shoulders in a stiff, neutral position. Pain is reproduced with active protraction or retraction of the shoulder, deep inspiration, and full elevation of the arm. Shrugging of the shoulder may also reproduce the pain. Coughing may be difficult, leading to inadequate pulmonary toilet in patients who have sustained trauma to the anterior chest wall. The manubriosternal joint may be tender to palpation. The patient may also complain of a clicking sensation with movement of the joint. With dislocation, a step-off will be obvious on visual inspection (see Fig. 2.1).

TESTING

Plain radiographs are indicated for all patients who present with pain thought to be emanating from the manubriosternal joint to rule out occult bony disorders, including tumor (Fig. 2.9). If trauma is present, radionuclide bone scanning may be useful to exclude occult fractures of the ribs or sternum. Based on the patient's clinical presentation, additional testing may be indicated, including a complete blood count, prostate-specific antigen level, erythrocyte sedimentation rate, and antinuclear antibody testing. Laboratory evaluation for

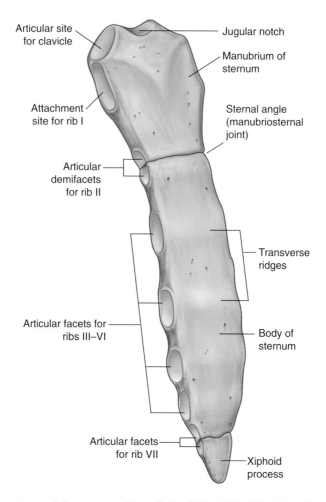

Fig. 2.4 The anatomy of the sternum. (From Drake R, Vogl W, Mitchell A. *Gray's Anatomy for Students*. ed. 4. Philadelphia: Churchill Livingstone; 2020 [Fig. 3-23].)

collagen vascular disease is indicated in patients suffering from manubriosternal joint pain if other joints are involved. Magnetic resonance imaging (MRI), ultrasound imaging, and/or computed tomography (CT) of the joint is indicated if joint instability, infection, or occult mass is suspected, or to further elucidate the cause of the pain (Figs. 2.10 and 2.11). The use of multidetector CT for patients presenting to the emergency department with acute chest pain has led to more rapid and accurate diagnosis of chest wall pain syndromes (see Fig. 2.6). The injection technique described later serves as both a diagnostic and a therapeutic maneuver (Fig. 2.12).

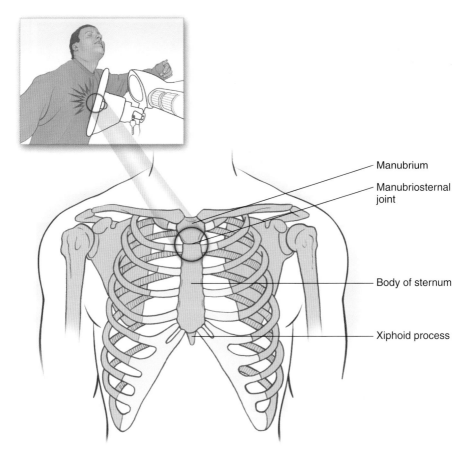

Fig. 2.5 The manubriosternal joint is susceptible to the development of arthritis. It is often traumatized during acceleration-deceleration injuries and blunt trauma to the chest. (From Waldman S. *Atlas of Common Pain Syndromes*. ed. 4. Philadelphia: Elsevier; 2019 [Fig. 62-1].)

DIFFERENTIAL DIAGNOSIS

As mentioned, the pain of manubriosternal syndrome is often mistaken for pain of cardiac origin, and it leads to visits to the emergency department and unnecessary cardiac workups. If trauma has occurred, manubriosternal syndrome may coexist with fractured ribs or fractures of the sternum itself, which can be missed on plain radiographs and may require radionuclide bone scanning for proper identification. Tietze syndrome, which is painful enlargement of the upper costochondral cartilage associated with viral infection, may be confused with manubriosternal syndrome.

Neuropathic pain involving the chest wall may also be confused or may coexist with manubriosternal syndrome. Examples of such neuropathic pain syndromes include diabetic polyneuropathies and acute herpes zoster

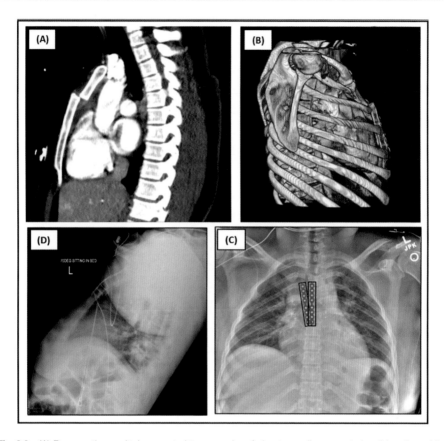

Fig. 2.6 (A) Preoperative sagittal computed tomography of chest revealing a posterior dislocation of the sternal body on the manubrium. (B) Preoperative sagittal three-dimensional reconstruction of chest. (C) Postoperative chest roentgenogram with sternal fixation plates and screws *(blue)*. (D) Postoperative lateral chest roentgenogram revealing stable sternum with fixation plate and screws. (From Sarkeshik AA, Jamal A, Perry PA. Manubriosternal joint dislocation due to blunt force trauma. *Trauma Case Rep.* 2019;21:100187 [Fig. 1]. ISSN 2352-6440, https://doi.org/10.1016/j.tcr.2019.100187, http://www.sciencedirect.com/science/article/pii/S2352644019300214.)

involving the thoracic nerves. Diseases of the structures of the mediastinum are possible and can be difficult to diagnose. Pathologic processes that inflame the pleura, such as pulmonary embolus, infection, and Bornholm disease, may also confuse the diagnosis and complicate treatment, as may undiagnosed systemic diseases that affect the manubriosternal joint (Fig. 2.13).

TREATMENT

Initial treatment of the pain and functional disability associated with manubriosternal syndrome includes a combination of nonsteroidal

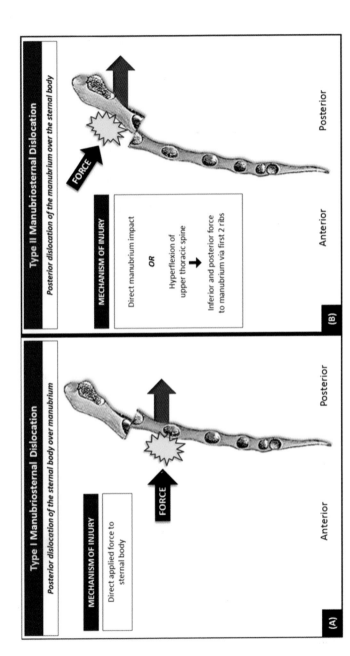

Fig. 2.7 Depiction of type I and type II manubriosternal joint dislocation injuries. (From Sarkeshik AA, Jamal A, Perry PA. Manubriosternal joint dislocation due to blunt force trauma. *Trauma Case Rep.* 2019;21:100187 [Fig. 2]. ISSN 2352-6440, https://doi.org/10.1016/j.tcr.2019.100187, http://www.sciencedirect.com/science/article/pii/S2352644019300214.)

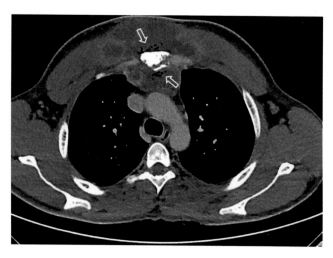

Fig. 2.8 Primary septic arthritis of the manubriosternal joint. Enhanced computed tomography axial image of the mass; note is made of the presence of small air bubbles related to suppurative soft tissue involvement *(arrows)*. (From Carnevale A, Righi R, Maniscalco P, et al. Primary septic arthritis of the manubriosternal joint in an immunocompetent young patient: a case report. *Radiol Case Rep.* 2017;12(4):682−685 [Fig. 3]. ISSN 1930-0433, https://doi.org/10.1016/j.radcr.2017.08.006, http://www.sciencedirect.com/science/article/pii/S1930043317302613.)

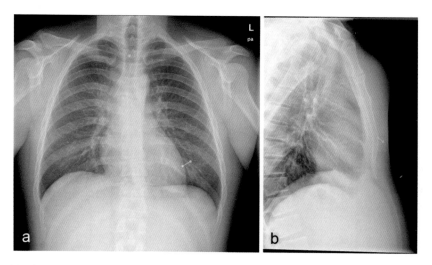

Fig. 2.9 Septic arthritis of the manubriosternal joint. (a) Posterior-anterior (PA) chest roentgenogram and (b) lateral *(L)* view of the sternum, showing a soft tissue swelling over the manubriosternal region; mild joint space widening and articular surfaces irregularity are noted. (From Carnevale A, Righi R, Maniscalco P, et al. Primary septic arthritis of the manubriosternal joint in an immunocompetent young patient: a case report. *Radiol Case Rep.* 2017;12(4):682−685 [Fig. 1]. ISSN 1930-0433, https://doi.org/10.1016/j.radcr.2017.08.006, http://www.sciencedirect.com/science/article/pii/S1930043317302613.)

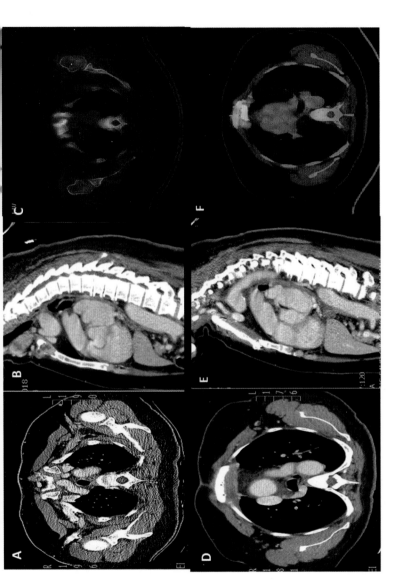

Fig. 2.10 (A, B) Computed tomography (CT) scan of the thorax, axial and sagittal views, showing manubrial metastasis. (C) Preoperative positron emission tomography (PET) scan of the thorax showing metastasis. (D, E) Postoperative CT scan showing reconstruction of the manubrium sternii with an MMS plate. (F) PET scan of the thorax after 2 years showing the methyl methacrylate marlex mesh plate (MMS) plate in good position and no recurrence. (From Chaudhry IUH, Cheema A, Aqeel C, et al. Radical resection and improvised manubriosternal reconstruction technique for solitary manubriosternal metastasis from papillary thyroid cancer. *Int J Surg Case Rep.* 2020;76:278–281 [Fig. 2]. ISSN 2210-2612, https://doi.org/10.1016/j.ijscr.2020.09.201, http://www.sciencedirect.com/science/article/pii/S2210261220308749.)

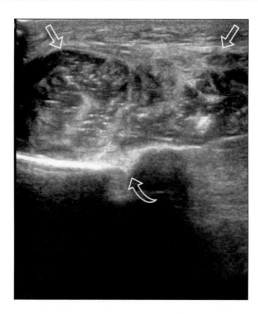

Fig. 2.11 Soft tissue ultrasonography, longitudinal plane, demonstrating a lobulated heteroge-neously hypoechoic mass *(straight arrows)* over the manubriosternal joint *(curved arrow)*. (From Carnevale A, Righi R, Maniscalco P, et al. Primary septic arthritis of the manubriosternal joint in an immunocompetent young patient: a case report. *Radiol Case Rep.* 2017;12(4):682−685 [Fig. 2]. ISSN 1930-0433, https://doi.org/10.1016/j.radcr.2017.08.006, http://www.sciencedirect.com/science/article/pii/S1930043317302613.)

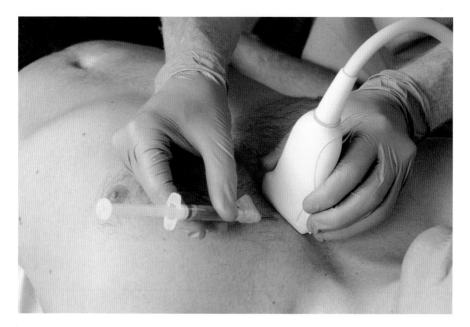

Fig. 2.12 Proper needle placement for out-of-plane ultrasound-guided injection of the manubriosternal joint.

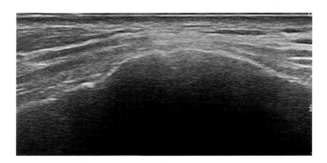

Fig. 2.13 Ultrasonographic image demonstrating ankylosis of the manubiosternal joint in longitudinal view. (From Verhoeven F, Sondag M, Chouk M, et al. Ultrasonographic involvement of the anterior chest wall in spondyloarthritis: factors associated with 5-years structural progression. A prospective study in 58 patients. *Joint Bone Spine.* 2020;87(4):321−325 [Fig. 1]. ISSN 1297-319X, https://doi.org/10.1016/j.jbspin.2020.02.008, http://www.sciencedirect.com/science/article/pii/S1297319X2030035X.)

antiinflammatory drugs or cyclooxygenase-2 inhibitors. The local application of heat and cold may also be beneficial. Use of an elastic rib belt may also provide symptomatic relief and protect the manubriosternal joint from additional trauma. For patients who do not respond to these treatment modalities, injection with local anesthetic and steroid may serve as both a diagnostic and therapeutic maneuver (see Fig. 2.12).

HIGH-YIELD TAKEAWAYS

- The patient is afebrile, making an acute infectious etiology unlikely.
- The patient's symptomatology is consistent with the classic clinical presentation of manubriosternal joint pain.
- Physical examination and testing should be focused on the identification of the other pathologic processes that may mimic the clinical diagnosis of manubriosternal joint dysfunction, in particular, malignant mediastinal tumors.
- X-ray, ultrasound, CT, and MRI of the chest wall may help confirm the diagnosis or identify unexpected causes of the patient's pain symptomatology.

Suggested Readings

Carnevale A, Righi R, Maniscalco P, et al. Primary septic arthritis of the manubriosternal joint in an immunocompetent young patient: a case report. *Radiol Case Rep.* 2017;12(4):682−685.

Kim DK, Kim KH, Park BK, et al. Atypical SAPHO syndrome with isolated manubriosternal inflammation: a multi-image demonstration. *PM&R.* 2016;8(7):716−717.

Lyons I, Saha S, Arulampalam T. Manubriosternal joint dislocation: an unusual risk of trampolining. *J Emerg Med*. 2010;39(5):596–598.

Sarkeshik AA, Jamal A, Perry PA. Manubriosternal joint dislocation due to blunt force trauma. *Trauma Case Rep*. 2019;21:100187.

Waldman SD. Arthritis and other abnormalities of the manubriosternal joint. In: *Waldman's Comprehensive Atlas of Diagnostic Ultrasound of Painful Conditions*. ed. 2. Philadelphia: Wolters Kluwer; 2016:519–525.

Waldman SD. Manubriosternal joint pain. In: *Atlas of Uncommon Pain Syndromes*. ed. 4. Philadelphia: Elsevier; 2021:233–236.

Waldman SD. Ultrasound-guided injection technique for the manubriosternal joint. In: *Waldman's Comprehensive Atlas of Ultrasound-Guided Pain Management Injection Techniques*. ed. 2. Philadelphia: Wolters Kluwer; 2020:595–599.

Doug Montgomery

A 38-Year-Old Male With Anterior Chest Wall Pain Made Worse by Bending

- Learn the common causes of xiphodynia.
- Develop an understanding of the anatomy of the xiphoid.
- Develop an understanding of the differential diagnosis of xiphodynia.
- Learn the clinical presentation of xiphodynia.
- Learn how to examine the xiphoid process.
- Learn how to examine the xiphoid and xiphisternal joint.
- Learn how to use physical examination to identify xiphodynia.
- Develop an understanding of the treatment options for xiphodynia.

Doug Montgomery

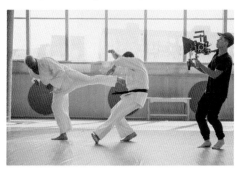

Doug Montgomery is a 36-year-old truck driver with the chief complaint of, "I can't exercise because my chest is killing me." Doug stated that ever since he took a hit to the chest during martial arts training, he has been suffering from severe chest wall pain. In spite of Advil, topical analgesic balm, and ice packs, the pain has persisted. He noted that the pain was made worse whenever he bent over or coughed. He went on to say, "I keep getting my days and nights mixed up because every time I roll over, it wakes me up." He said that he was afraid he would fall asleep while driving and kill himself or somebody else. I asked Doug if he ever had anything like this in the past, and he said, "Not really, just the usual back pain after driving over the road all day." I asked if he was experiencing any other symptoms associated with the chest pain, such as sweating, palpitations, or pain into the jaw or left arm, and he shook his head no. I asked Doug about any fever, chills, or other constitutional symptoms, such as weight loss or night sweats, and he again shook his head no.

I then asked Doug to point with one finger to show me where it hurt the most. He pointed to the area just above his xiphoid process.

On physical examination, Doug was afebrile. His respirations were 16, his pulse was 66 and regular, and his blood pressure was 112/68. Doug's head, eyes, ears, nose, throat (HEENT) exam was normal, as was his cardiopulmonary examination. Examination of the thyroid gland was normal and well muscled. His abdominal examination revealed no abnormal mass or organomegaly. There was no costovertebral angle (CVA) tenderness. There was no peripheral edema. His low back examination was unremarkable. Visual inspection of the anterior chest wall revealed visual prominence of the xiphoid process (Fig. 3.1). There was no rubor, ecchymosis, or obvious infection. Palpation of the xiphoid process caused Doug to cry out in pain (Fig. 3.2). A careful neurologic examination of the upper extremities was completely normal. Deep tendon reflexes were normal.

Key Clinical Points—What's Important and What's Not

THE HISTORY

■ History of the onset of xiphoid pain following a kick to the chest during martial arts training

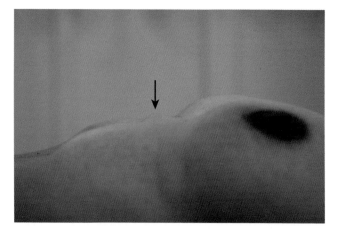

Fig. 3.1 Visual prominence of the xyphoid process. (From Maigne J-Y, Vareli M, Rousset P, et al. Xiphodynia and prominence of the xyphoid process: value of xiphosternal angle measurement—three case reports. *Joint Bone Spine*. 2010;77:474—476.)

- No numbness
- No weakness
- No history of previous chest wall trauma or chest pain
- No fever or chills

THE PHYSICAL EXAMINATION

- Patient is afebrile
- Normal cardiovascular examination
- Pain on palpation of the xiphoid process (see Fig. 3.2)

OTHER FINDINGS OF NOTE

- Normal HEENT examination
- Normal pulmonary examination
- Normal abdominal examination
- No peripheral edema
- Normal upper extremity neurologic examination, motor and sensory examination

 What Tests Would You Like to Order?

The following tests were ordered:
- Plain radiographs of the sternum and xiphoid process
- Ultrasound of the xiphisternal joint

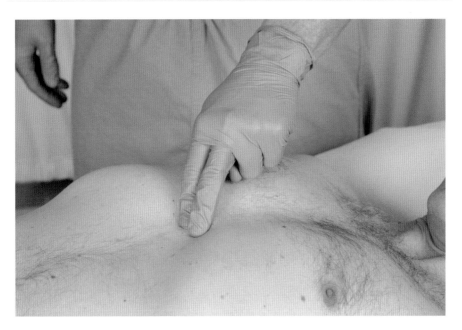

Fig. 3.2 Palpation of the xiphoid process.

TEST RESULTS

The plain radiographs of the xiphoid revealed that the xiphoid process projected anteriorly at an angle of 133 degrees from the sternal body (Fig. 3.3).

Ultrasound examination of the right xiphisternal joint revealed no obvious abnormality (Fig. 3.4).

Clinical Correlation—Putting It All Together

What is the diagnosis?
- Xiphodynia

The Science Behind the Diagnosis
ANATOMY

The xiphoid process articulates with the sternum via the xiphisternal joint (Fig. 3.5). The xiphoid process is a plate of cartilaginous bone that becomes calcified in early adulthood. The xiphisternal joint is strengthened by ligaments but can be subluxed or dislocated by blunt trauma to the anterior chest.

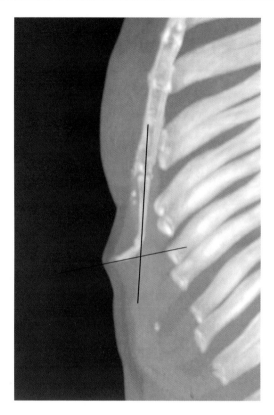

Fig. 3.3 Lateral radiograph of the xiphoid. Note the anterior angulation of the tip of the xyphoid. (From Maigne J-Y, Vareli M, Rousset P, et al. Xiphodynia and prominence of the xyphoid process: value of xiphosternal angle measurement—three case reports. *Joint Bone Spine*. 2010;77:474–476.)

The xiphisternal joint is innervated by the T4-T7 intercostal nerves and by the phrenic nerve. It is thought that this innervation by the phrenic nerve is responsible for the referred pain associated with xiphodynia syndrome. Posterior to the xiphisternal joint are the structures of the mediastinum. These structures are susceptible to needle-induced trauma if the needle is placed too deeply. The pleural space may be entered if the needle is placed too deeply and laterally, and pneumothorax may result.

CLINICAL SYNDROME

An uncommon cause of anterior chest wall pain, xiphodynia is often misdiagnosed as pain of cardiac or upper abdominal origin. Xiphodynia syndrome is a constellation of symptoms consisting of severe intermittent anterior chest wall pain in the region of the xiphoid process that worsens with overeating, stooping, and bending. The patient may report a nauseated feeling associated with the

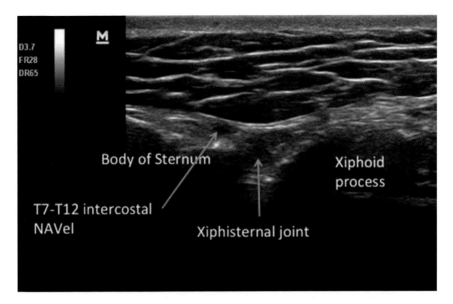

Fig. 3.4 Longitudinal ultrasound image of the xiphisternal joint.

pain of xiphodynia syndrome. This xiphisternal joint seems to serve as the nidus of pain for xiphodynia syndrome.

The xiphisternal joint is often traumatized during acceleration-deceleration injuries and blunt trauma to the chest. With severe trauma, the joint may sublux or dislocate. The xiphisternal joint also is susceptible to the development of arthritis, including osteoarthritis, rheumatoid arthritis, ankylosing spondylitis, Reiter syndrome, and psoriatic arthritis. The joint is subject to invasion by tumor from either primary malignancies, including thymoma, or metastatic disease.

SIGNS AND SYMPTOMS

Physical examination reveals that the pain of xiphodynia syndrome is reproduced with palpation or traction on the xiphoid (see Fig. 3.2). The xiphisternal joint may feel swollen (Fig. 3.6). Stooping or bending may reproduce the pain. Coughing may be difficult, and this may lead to inadequate pulmonary toilet in patients who have sustained trauma to the anterior chest wall. The xiphisternal joint and adjacent intercostal muscles also may be tender to palpation. The patient may report a clicking sensation with movement of the joint. Furthermore, patients with a prominent xiphoid process whose visual inspection indicates an xiphisternal angle of less than 160 degrees are more prone to the development of xiphodynia (Fig. 3.7).

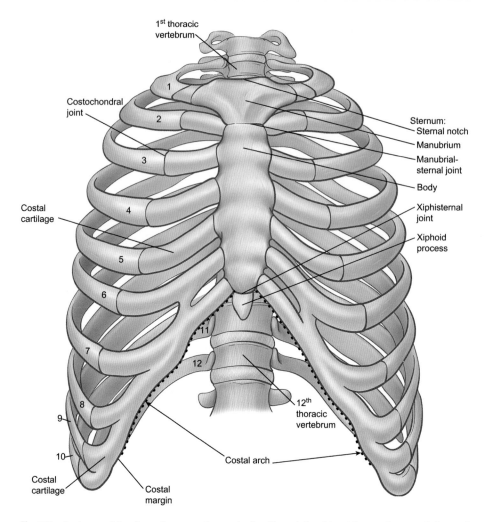

Fig. 3.5 Anatomy of the thoracic cage, demonstrating the relationship of the cartilage and ribs and major joints. (From Graeber GM, Nazim M. The anatomy of the ribs and the sternum and their relationship to chest wall structure and function. *Thorac Surg Clin*. 2007;17(4):473–489 [Fig. 6]. ISSN 1547-4127, https://doi.org/10.1016/j.thorsurg.2006.12.010, http://www.sciencedirect.com/science/article/pii/S154741270600106X.)

TESTING

Plain radiographs are indicated in all patients with pain thought to be emanating from the xiphisternal joint to rule out occult bony pathologic conditions, including tumor (see Fig. 3.4). Based on the patient's clinical presentation, additional tests (complete blood cell count, prostate-specific antigen level, erythrocyte sedimentation rate, and antinuclear antibody testing) may be

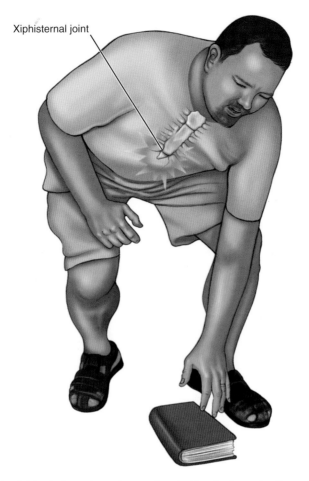

Xiphisternal joint

Fig. 3.6 The pain of xiphodynia syndrome is reproduced with palpation or traction on the xiphoid. The xiphisternal joint may feel swollen. Stooping or bending may reproduce the pain. (From Waldman S. *Atlas of Uncommon Pain Syndromes*. ed. 4. Philadelphia: Elsevier; 2020 [Fig. 70-1].)

indicated. Computed tomography (CT), ultrasound imaging, or magnetic resonance imaging (MRI) of the joint is indicated if joint instability or an occult mass is suspected (Figs. 3.8, 3.9, and 3.10). The injection of the xiphisternal joint with local anesthetic and steroid serves as a diagnostic and therapeutic maneuver.

DIFFERENTIAL DIAGNOSIS

As with costochondritis, costosternal joint pain, devil's grip, Tietze syndrome, and rib fractures, many patients with xiphodynia first seek medical attention because they believe they are having a heart attack.

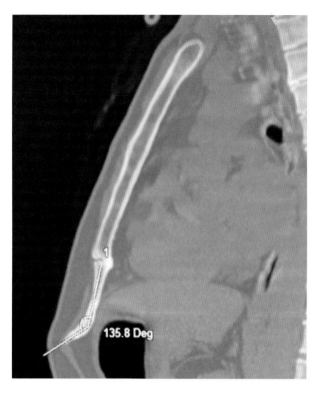

Fig. 3.7 Sagittal computed tomography scan in a bone window showing a developed xiphoid appendage protruding under the skin with a xiphosternal angle of 135.8 degrees. (From Doulhousne H, Toufga Z, Roukhsi R, et al. La xiphodynie: une douleur peu commune. *J d'imagerie diagn et interv*. 2020;3(2):139-140 [Fig. 1]. ISSN 2543-3431, https://doi.org/10.1016/j.jidi.2019.11.005, http://www.sciencedirect.com/science/article/pii/S2543343119301952.)

Patients also may believe they have ulcer or gallbladder disease. In contrast to most other causes of pain involving the chest wall that are musculoskeletal or neuropathic in origin, the pain of devil's grip results from infection. The constitutional symptoms associated with devil's grip may lead the clinician to consider pneumonia, empyema, and occasionally pulmonary embolus as the most likely diagnosis.

TREATMENT

Initial treatment of xiphodynia should include a combination of simple analgesics and nonsteroidal antiinflammatory drugs or cyclooxygenase-2 inhibitors. If these medications do not control the patient's symptoms adequately, opioid analgesics may be added during the period of acute pain. Local application of heat and cold may be beneficial to provide symptomatic relief of the pain of

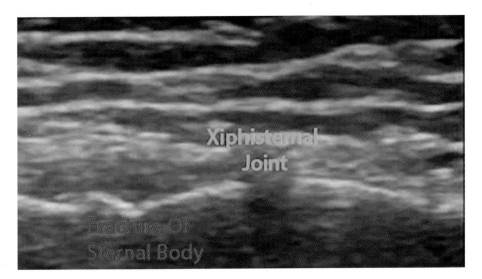

Fig. 3.8 Longitudinal ultrasound image of the xiphisternal joint in a patient with xiphidynia, demonstrating an unsuspected fracture of the sternal body from a seatbelt injury.

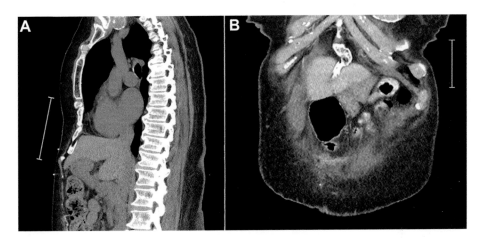

Fig. 3.9 Computed tomographic scans showing heterotopic ossification of the xyphoid in a patient with previous xiphid fractures from chest compressions during cardiopulmonary resuscitation. (A) Sagittal; (B) coronal. (From Vu TND, Aho JM, Puig CA, et al. Heterotopic ossification of the xiphoid after chest compressions. *Ann Thorac Surg.* 2019;108:e347–e348 [Fig. 1]. ISSN 0003-4975, https://doi.org/10.1016/j.athoracsur.2019.03.110, http://www.sciencedirect.com/science/article/pii/S000349 7519306897.)

xiphodynia. The use of an elastic rib belt may help provide symptomatic relief in some patients. For patients who do not respond to these treatment modalities, the injection of the xiphisternal joint using a local anesthetic and steroid may be a reasonable next step (Fig. 3.11).

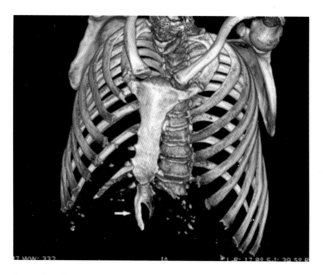

Fig. 3.10 Three-dimensional computerized tomographic reconstruction of the thoracic cage in a patient with xiphodynia. Note the curved, bifid xiphoid thought to be responsible for the patient's pain symptomatology. (From Doulhousne H, Toufga Z, Roukhsi R, et al. La xiphodynie: une douleur peu commune. *J d'imag diagn et interv*. 2020;3(2):139–140 [Fig. 2]. ISSN 2543-3431, https://doi.org/10.1016/j.jidi.2019.11.005, http://www.sciencedirect.com/science/article/pii/S2543343119301952.)

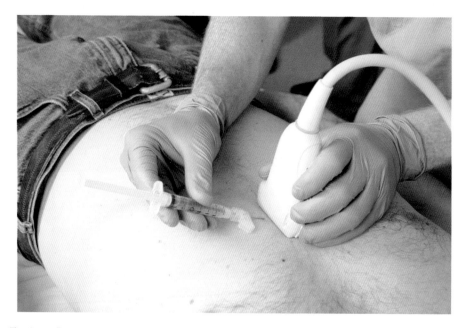

Fig. 3.11 Proper needle placement for out-of-plane ultrasound-guided injection of the xiphisternal joint.

HIGH-YIELD TAKEAWAYS

- The patient is afebrile, making an acute infectious etiology unlikely.
- The patient's symptomatology began after acute trauma to the chest wall from a kick to the sternum during martial arts practice.
- Physical examination and testing should be focused on the identification of the various causes of xiphodynia.
- The patient exhibits physical examination findings that are highly suggestive of xiphodynia.
- The patient's symptoms are unilateral, suggestive of a local process rather than a systemic inflammatory process.
- Plain radiographs and CT will provide high-yield information regarding the bony abnormalities, but ultrasound imaging and MRI will be more useful in identifying soft tissue pathology that may be responsible for xiphoidynia.

Suggested Readings

Maigne J-Y, Vareli M, Rousset P, et al. Xiphodynia and prominence of the xyphoid process. Value of xiphosternal angle measurement: three case reports. *Joint Bone Spine*. 2010;77(5):474–476.

Vu TND, Aho JM, Puig CA, et al. Heterotopic ossification of the xiphoid after chest compressions. *Ann Thorac Surg*. 2019;108(6):e347–e348.

Waldman SD. Arthritis and other abnormalities of the xiphisternal joint. In: *Waldman's Comprehensive Atlas of Diagnostic Ultrasound of Painful Conditions*. ed. 2. Philadelphia: Wolters Kluwer; 2016:526–529.

Waldman SD. Ultrasound-guided injection technique for the xiphisternal joint. In: *Waldman's Comprehensive Atlas of Ultrasound-Guided Pain Management Injection Techniques*. ed. 2. Philadelphia: Wolters Kluwer; 2020:600–605.

Waldman SD. Xiphodynia. In: *Atlas of Uncommon Pain Syndromes*. ed. 4. Philadelphia: Elsevier; 2019:237–239.

4

Jill St. John, BSN

A 25-Year-Old Female With Chest Wall Pain and a Cold

- Learn the common causes of chest wall pain.
- Develop an understanding of the unique anatomy of the chest wall.
- Develop an understanding of the anatomy of the costosternal joint.
- Develop an understanding of the causes of Tietze syndrome.
- Develop an understanding of the differential diagnosis of Tietze syndrome.
- Learn the clinical presentation of Tietze syndrome.
- Learn how to examine the chest wall.
- Learn how to use physical examination to identify Tietze syndrome.
- Develop an understanding of the treatment options for Tietze syndrome.

Jill St. John

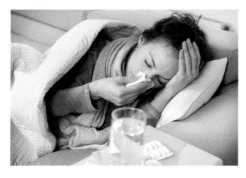

Jill St. John is a 25-year-old emergency department (ED) nurse with the chief complaint of, "I have a bad cold and it hurts to cough." Jill stated that she picked up an upper respiratory tract infection while working in the ED, and over the past 4 days, she began experiencing severe pain and swelling at the top of her sternum. She denied any antecedent trauma but noted that she was having trouble coughing because of the pain. "Doctor, I am afraid I am going to get pneumonia. It hurts so bad to cough that I am having trouble clearing secretions. It really hurts when I raise my arms. I know that I look a mess, but it just hurts too much to brush out my hair. I've been taking Motrin around the clock, but the pain really isn't a lot better. This is about the worst cold I have ever had, but the pain is why I came to see you. I wonder if I separated a cartilage from all the coughing?" I asked Jill if she ever had any pain in her anterior chest before, and she shook her head no.

She said that on the first day when she was coming down with her cold that she might have had a mild fever, but she denied chills or other constitutional symptoms. "I knew it was just a cold, so I figured I would get better on my own, but then this pain started. I've already missed three shifts at work, and we are really shorthanded." I asked Jill what made her pain better, and she said that a heating pad helped the pain a little, but the Motrin wasn't doing much more than upsetting her stomach. She noted that between being congested and having pain in the chest wall, she wasn't getting much sleep.

I asked Jill about any antecedent chest wall trauma, and she shook her head no. She volunteered, "Doctor, I am never sick, but this has really knocked me on my butt. I feel like the upper part of my sternum is swollen, and it is very tender when I palpate it. Something isn't right. Like I said, I may have separated a cartilage or something."

I asked Jill to point with one finger to show me where it hurt the most. She pointed to the left side of her sternum at about the third costosternal cartilage. "Doctor, it really hurts all around this area, and when I cough, it's pretty rough."

On physical examination, Jill was afebrile. Her respirations were 16, and her pulse was 79 and regular. Her oxygen saturation on room air was 98. Her blood pressure was 120/70. Jill's head, eyes, ears, nose, throat (HEENT) exam was consistent with a bad upper respiratory tract infection. Her nares were red, and she looked miserable. In spite of her upper respiratory symptoms, her lungs were clear, although I could hear some upper airway secretions that cleared when

I had Jill cough. Her cardiac examination was normal. Her thyroid was normal. Her abdominal examination revealed no abnormal mass or organomegaly. There was no costovertebral angle (CVA) tenderness. There was no peripheral edema. Her low back examination was unremarkable. Visual inspection of the chest wall revealed there was swelling over the second and third costosternal joints on the right consistent with a positive swollen costosternal joint sign. Palpation of the affected costosternal joints revealed that they felt a little warm. There was marked tenderness to palpation of the area overlying the right second and third intercostal joints. The examination of the remainder of her chest wall was normal, as was examination of her other major joints. A careful neurologic examination of the upper extremities revealed no evidence of peripheral neuropathy or entrapment neuropathy. Deep tendon reflexes were normal.

Key Clinical Points—What's Important and What's Not

THE HISTORY

- History of onset of anterior chest wall pain associated with an upper respiratory tract infection
- No history of previous significant chest wall pain
- Minimal fever and no chills or other constitutional symptoms
- Severe chest wall pain when coughing
- Pain to palpation of the upper costosternal cartilages
- Swelling of the upper costosternal cartilages noted by patient
- Exacerbation of pain when elevating the upper extremities

THE PHYSICAL EXAMINATION

- Patient is afebrile
- Point tenderness to palpation of the second and third costosternal cartilage on the right
- Swelling of the second and third costosternal cartilage on the right
- Warmth over the second and third costosternal cartilage on the right
- No evidence of pneumonia
- Positive swollen costosternal joint sign

OTHER FINDINGS OF NOTE

- Normal HEENT examination
- Normal cardiovascular examination
- Normal pulmonary examination
- Normal abdominal examination

- No peripheral edema
- Normal neurologic examination
- Examination of major joints normal

What Tests Would You Like to Order?

The following test was ordered:
- Plain radiographs of the sternum

TEST RESULTS

The plain radiographs of the sternum revealed mild swelling of the second and third costosternal joints on the right.

Clinical Correlation—Putting It All Together

What is the diagnosis?
- Tietze syndrome

The Science Behind the Diagnosis

ANATOMY

The cartilage of the true ribs articulates with the sternum via the costosternal joints (Fig. 4.1). The cartilage of the first rib articulates directly with the manubrium of the sternum and is a synarthrodial joint that allows a limited gliding movement. The cartilage of the second through sixth ribs articulates with the body of the sternum via true arthrodial joints. These joints are surrounded by a thin articular capsule. The costosternal joints are strengthened by ligaments but can be subluxed or dislocated by blunt trauma to the anterior chest. Posterior to the costosternal joint are the structures of the mediastinum. These structures are susceptible to needle-induced trauma if the needle is placed too deeply. The pleural space may be entered if the needle is placed too deeply and laterally, and pneumothorax may result (Fig. 4.2).

CLINICAL SYNDROME

Tietze syndrome is a frequent cause of chest wall pain. Distinct from the more common costosternal syndrome, Tietze syndrome was first described in 1921 and is characterized by acute, painful swelling of the costal cartilage. In fact,

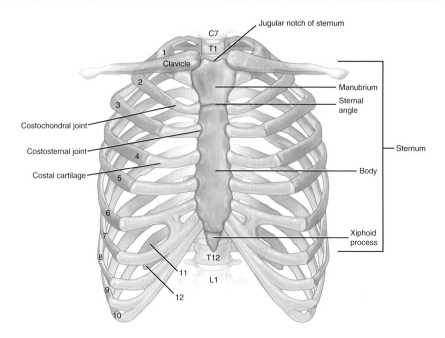

Fig. 4.1 The anatomy of the chest wall. (From Waldman S. *Atlas of Pain Management Injection Techniques*. ed. 4. St. Louis: Elsevier; 2017 [Fig. 99-3].)

painful swelling of the second and third costochondral joints is the sine qua non of Tietze syndrome (Fig. 4.3); such swelling is absent in costosternal syndrome. Also distinguishing the two syndromes is the age of onset. Whereas costosternal syndrome usually occurs no earlier than the fourth decade of life, Tietze syndrome is a disease of the second and third decades. The onset is acute and is often associated with a concurrent viral infection of the respiratory tract. Investigators have postulated that microtrauma to the costosternal joints from severe coughing or heavy labor may be the cause of Tietze syndrome.

SIGNS AND SYMPTOMS

Physical examination reveals that patients suffering from Tietze syndrome vigorously attempt to splint the joints by keeping the shoulders in a stiff, neutral position. Pain is reproduced with active protraction or retraction of the shoulder, deep inspiration, and full elevation of the arm. Shrugging of the shoulder may also reproduce the pain. Coughing may be difficult, leading to inadequate pulmonary toilet in some patients. The costosternal joints, especially the second and third, are swollen and exquisitely tender to palpation (Fig. 4.4). This swollen costochondral joint sign is pathognomonic for Tietze

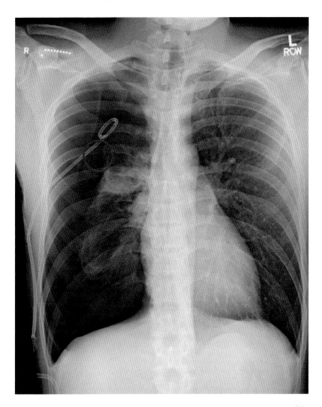

Fig. 4.2 X-ray demonstrating right-sided pneumothorax *(red circle)*. (From Segraves JM, Dulohery MM. Primary spontaneous pneumothorax due to high bleb burden. *Respir Med Case Rep.* 2016;19:109-111 [Fig. 2]. ISSN 2213-0071, https://doi.org/10.1016/j.rmcr.2016.08.007, http://www. sciencedirect.com/science/article/pii/S2213007116300806.)

syndrome (Fig. 4.5). The adjacent intercostal muscles may also be tender to palpation. The patient may complain of a clicking sensation with movement of the joint.

TESTING

Plain radiographs are indicated for all patients who present with pain thought to be emanating from the costosternal joints to rule out occult bony disorders, including tumor (Fig. 4.6). If trauma is present, radionuclide bone scanning should be considered to exclude occult fractures of the ribs or sternum. Based on the patient's clinical presentation, additional testing may be indicated, including a complete blood count, prostate-specific antigen level, erythrocyte sedimentation rate, and antinuclear antibody testing. Laboratory evaluation for collagen vascular disease is

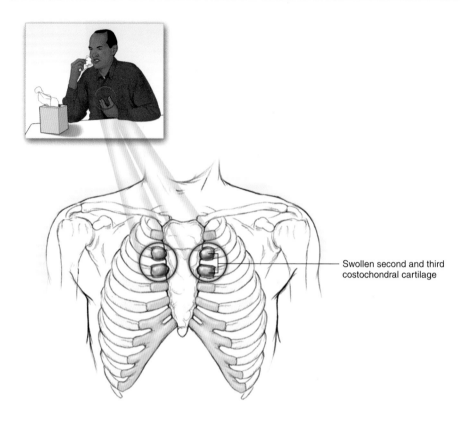

Swollen second and third
costochondral cartilage

Fig. 4.3 Swelling of the second and third costochondral joints is pathognomonic of Tietze syndrome. (From Waldman S. *Atlas of Common Pain Syndromes*. ed. 4. Philadelphia: Elsevier; 2019 [Fig. 65-1].)

indicated in patients suffering from costosternal joint pain if other joints are involved. Magnetic resonance imaging (MRI), computed tomography (CT), and ultrasound imaging of the joints are indicated if joint instability or occult mass is suspected, or to confirm the diagnosis (Figs. 4.7 and 4.8). Injection of the affected costosternal joints serves as both a diagnostic and a therapeutic maneuver (Fig. 4.9).

DIFFERENTIAL DIAGNOSIS

Many other painful conditions that affect the costosternal joints are much more common than Tietze syndrome. For instance, the costosternal joints are susceptible to osteoarthritis, rheumatoid arthritis, ankylosing spondylitis, Reiter syndrome, and psoriatic arthritis (Fig. 4.10). The joints are often traumatized during

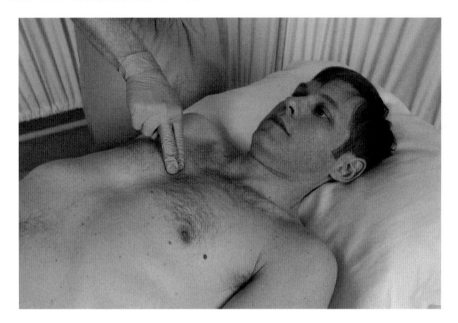

Fig. 4.4   Palpation of the costosternal joint.

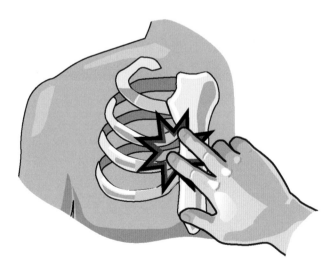

Fig. 4.5   The swollen costosternal sign for Tietze sign. (From Waldman S. *Physical Diagnosis of Pain: An Atlas of Signs and Symptoms*. ed. 4. Philadelphia: Elsevier; 2021 [Fig. 144-2].)

acceleration-deceleration injuries and blunt trauma to the chest; with severe trauma, the joints may subluxate or dislocate. Overuse or misuse can result in acute inflammation of the costosternal joint, which can be quite debilitating. The

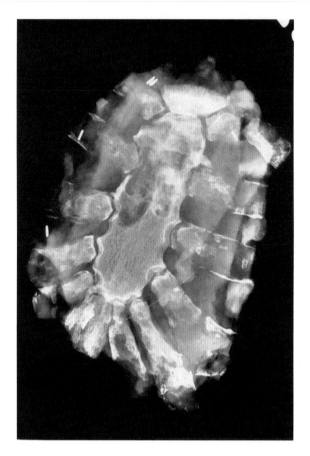

Fig. 4.6 Radiograph of resected chest wall in 54-year-old man with low-grade chondrosarcoma of body of sternum. Resection included body, xiphoid process, and lower portion of manubrium. Tumor is clearly seen in upper part of body of sternum. (From Martini N, Huvos AG, Burt ME, et al. Predictors of survival in malignant tumors of the sternum. *J Thorac Cardiovasc Surg.* 1996;111(1):96–106 [Fig. 3]. ISSN 0022-5223, https://doi.org/10.1016/S0022-5223(96)70405-1, http://www.sciencedirect.com/science/article/pii/S0022522396704051.)

joints are also subject to invasion by tumor from primary malignant tumors, including thymoma, or from metastatic disease.

TREATMENT

Initial treatment of the pain and functional disability associated with Tietze syndrome includes nonsteroidal antiinflammatory drugs (NSAIDs) or cyclooxygenase-2 inhibitors. The local application of heat and cold may also be beneficial. Use of an

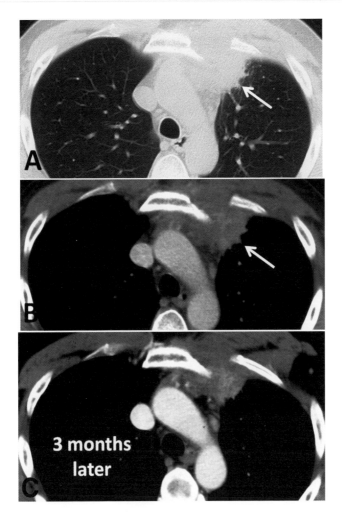

Fig. 4.7 Computed tomography (CT) scan of a patient with anterior chest wall pain thought to be Tietze syndrome. CT scanning of anterior upper mediastinal mass after iodinated contrast administration. Lung window (A). Mediastinum window (B) shows inhomogeneous contrast enhancement of the mass. Enhanced multidetector CT follow-up after 3 months (C) shows decrease in volume of mediastinal mass. (From De Filippo M, Albini A, Castaldi V, et al. MRI findings of Tietze's syndrome mimicking mediastinal malignancy on MDCT. *Eur J Radiol Extra.* 2008;65(1):33—35 [Fig. 1]. ISSN 1571-4675, https://doi.org/10.1016/j.ejrex.2007.10.006, http://www.sciencedirect.com/science/article/pii/S1571467507000892.)

elastic rib belt may provide symptomatic relief and protect the costosternal joints from additional trauma. For patients who do not respond to these treatment modalities, injection using local anesthetic and steroid is a reasonable next step (see Fig. 4.9).

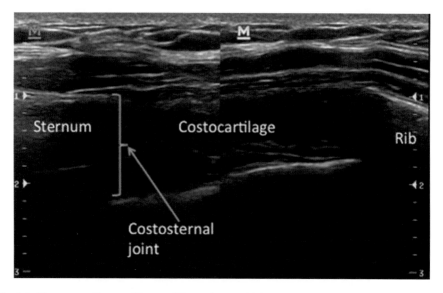

Fig. 4.8   Transverse ultrasound image of the costosternal joint.

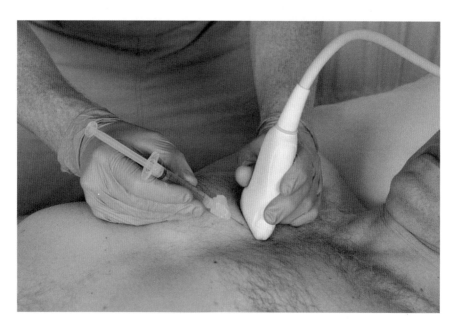

Fig. 4.9   Proper needle placement for ultrasound-guided injection of the costosternal joint for Tieitze syndrome.

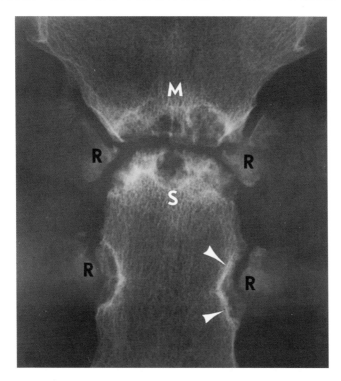

Fig. 4.10 Abnormalities of manubriosternal and sternocostal joints in rheumatoid arthritis. Radiograph of a sternum from a cadaver with rheumatoid arthritis shows large erosions of the articular surface of both the manubrium *(M)* and the body of the sternum *(S)*. Subtle irregularities of the second and third sternocostal joints are evident, most prominently in the sternal facet of the left third sternocostal joint *(arrowheads)*. R, Ossified costal cartilage. (From Resnick D. *Diagnosis of Bone and Joint Disorders*. ed. 4. Philadelphia: Saunders; 2002:854.)

Physical modalities, including local heat and gentle range-of-motion exercises, should be introduced several days after the patient undergoes injection for Tietze syndrome. Vigorous exercises should be avoided because they will exacerbate the patient's symptoms. Simple analgesics and NSAIDs may be used concurrently with this injection technique.

HIGH-YIELD TAKEAWAYS

- The patient is afebrile, making an acute infectious etiology (e.g., septic arthritis) unlikely.
- The patient's symptomatology is clinically consistent with Tietze syndrome.

(Continued)

- Physical examination and testing should be focused on the identification of infection, tumor, and other pathologic processes that may mimic Tietze syndrome.
- The patient has swelling of the second and third costosternal joints.
- The patient has point tenderness over the second and third costosternal joints.
- The patient's symptoms are localized, which is more suggestive of a local process than a systemic polyarthropathy.
- The patient has a positive swollen costosternal joint sign.
- Plain radiographs will provide high-yield information regarding the bony contents of the joint, but ultrasound imaging and MRI will be more useful in identifying soft tissue pathology.

Suggested Readings

Gologorsky R, Hornik B, Velotta J. Surgical management of medically refractory Tietze syndrome. *Ann Thorac Surg.* 2017;104(6):e443—e445.

Hanak JA. Tietze syndrome. In: Frontera WR, Silver JK, Rizzo TD, eds. *Essentials of Physical Medicine and Rehabilitation.* ed. 4. Philadelphia: Elsevier; 2020:640—645.

Waldman SD. Arthritis and other abnormalities of the costosternal joint. In: *Waldman's Comprehensive Atlas of Diagnostic Ultrasound of Painful Conditions.* ed. 4. Philadelphia: Wolters Kluwer; 2016:513—518.

Waldman SD. The swollen costosternal joint sign for Tietze syndrome. In: *Physical Diagnosis of Pain: An Atlas of Signs and Symptoms.* ed. 4. Philadelphia: Elsevier; 2021:228—229.

Waldman SD. Tietze's syndrome. In: *Atlas of Common Pain Syndromes.* ed. 4. Philadelphia: Elsevier; 2019:254—256.

Waldman SD. Ultrasound-guided injection technique for costosternal joint pain. In: *Waldman's Comprehensive Atlas of Ultrasound-Guided Pain Management Injection Techniques.* ed. 2. Philadelphia: Wolters Kluwer; 2020:591—594.

Val Rider

A 29-Year-Old Female With Persistent Burning Rib Pain Following a Rib Fracture

- Learn the common causes of chest wall pain.
- Develop an understanding of the unique anatomy of the chest wall.
- Develop an understanding of the anatomy of the intercostal nerve.
- Develop an understanding of the causes of intercostal neuralgia.
- Develop an understanding of the differential diagnosis of intercostal neuralgia.
- Learn the clinical presentation of intercostal neuralgia.
- Learn how to examine the chest wall.
- Learn how to use physical examination to identify intercostal neuralgia.
- Develop an understanding of the treatment options for intercostal neuralgia.

Val Rider

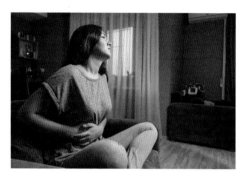

Val Rider is a 29-year-old buyer for a local market with the chief complaint of, "Ever since I broke my ribs, my chest has been killing me." Val stated that about 4 months ago, she had a bike accident and broke a couple of ribs. The ribs gradually healed, but she has been left with persistent, burning pain over the area of the broken ribs. Val noted that in spite of trying Advil, a rib belt, and a heating pad, the pain "just isn't getting any better." More recently, Val began noticing an area of numbness in the skin overlying the painful area. "Doctor, I know that this will sound crazy, but the area where my broken ribs were hurts and feels funny, kind of a numb feeling at the same time. Is this all in my head? This just doesn't make any sense." I said that it was unlikely it was all in her head and that together, we would figure out what was causing her symptoms. I asked Val if she had ever experienced anything like this in the past, and she said no. I asked whether she had any rash in the area of the broken ribs, and she shook her head and said absolutely not. She denied any fever, chills, or other constitutional symptoms associated with her pain. Her last period was 10 days ago. I asked Val what made her pain better, and she said that sometimes a lidocaine patch provided some relief, but they were so expensive that she only used them when the pain was really bad. I asked if she had tried ice or heat, and she said she tried a heating pad but thought it made the pain worse. She denied significant sleep disturbance. I asked if any specific movement made the pain worse, and she said, "Since the ribs healed, moving or lying on the area doesn't seem to change things one way or the other." I asked Val about any antecedent rib or chest wall trauma, and she shook her head no. She also denied any recent surgery.

I asked Val to point with one finger to show me where it hurt the most. She pointed to the top of the area overlying the 10th, 11th, and 12th ribs on the right, and said, "Doctor, it really seems to be this whole area over where I broke my ribs. Such a stupid accident, lucky I didn't get killed. That idiot opened his car door right in front of me, and I ran right into it. I went flying over the handlebars, my bike was totaled, and so were my ribs." Val poked her ribs on the right and said, "It's like the ribs that were broken hurt, but they really don't. Even when I really push on them, this whole area feels like a piece of wood. It just doesn't feel right, just kinda dead. This whole thing is just nuts."

On physical examination, Val was afebrile. Her respirations were 16, and her pulse was 68 and regular. Her blood pressure was 118/70. Val's head, eyes, ears, nose, throat (HEENT) exam was normal, as was her cardiopulmonary examination. Her thyroid was normal. Her abdominal examination revealed no abnormal mass or organomegaly. There was no costovertebral angle (CVA) tenderness. There was no peripheral edema. Her low back examination was unremarkable. Visual inspection of the right chest wall revealed no evidence of herpes zoster or obvious bony deformity. There was really no tenderness to palpation of the area overlying the right lower anterolateral chest wall, but careful sensory testing revealed decreased sensation from the posterior axillary line to the anterior chest wall and subcostal area in the distribution of the right 10th and 11th intercostal and subcostal nerves. Examinations of the left chest wall, dorsal spine, and other major joints were unremarkable. A careful neurologic examination revealed that other than the sensory deficit of the right intercostal nerves, there was no evidence of peripheral neuropathy. Deep tendon reflexes were normal.

Key Clinical Points—What's Important and What's Not

THE HISTORY

- History of acute trauma with associated broken ribs
- No history of previous significant chest wall pain
- No fever or chills
- Persistent burning right lower chest wall pain with associated numbness
- Movement does not exacerbate the pain
- No history of rash in the area of pain and numbness

THE PHYSICAL EXAMINATION

- Patient is afebrile
- Minimal tenderness to palpation of the right 10th, 11th, and 12th ribs
- Decreased sensation in the distribution of the right 10th and 11th intercostal and subcostal nerves
- No evidence of infection

OTHER FINDINGS OF NOTE

- Normal HEENT examination
- Normal cardiovascular examination
- Normal pulmonary examination
- Normal abdominal examination
- No peripheral edema

- Normal upper extremity neurologic examination, motor and sensory examination with exception of numbness in the distribution of the right 10th and 11th intercostal and subcostal nerves
- Examination of major joints normal

 ## What Tests Would You Like to Order?

The following tests were ordered:
- Plain radiographs of the chest with right lower rib details
- Computed tomography (CT) scan of the chest
- Electromyography (EMG) and nerve conduction velocity testing of the right 10th and 11th intercostal and subcostal nerves

TEST RESULTS

The plain radiographs of the right chest were normal.

The radiographs of the right 10th, 11th, and 12th ribs revealed healing rib fractures.

Findings from the EMG and nerve conduction tests of the right 10th and 11th intercostal and subcostal nerves were consistent with intercostal neuralgia.

 ## Clinical Correlation—Putting It All Together

What is the diagnosis?
- Intercostal neuralgia

The Science Behind the Diagnosis
ANATOMY

The intercostal nerves arise from the anterior division of the thoracic paravertebral nerve. A typical intercostal nerve has four major branches (Fig. 5.1). The first branch is the unmyelinated postganglionic fibers of the gray rami communicantes, which interface with the sympathetic chain. The second branch is the posterior cutaneous branch, which innervates the muscles and skin of the paraspinal area. The third branch is the lateral cutaneous division, which arises in the anterior axillary line and provides the majority of the cutaneous innervation of the chest and abdominal wall. The fourth branch is the anterior cutaneous branch, which supplies innervation to the midline of the chest and abdominal wall (see Fig. 5.1). The anterior cutaneous branch pierces the fascia of the abdominal wall at the lateral border of the rectus abdominis muscle (Fig. 5.2). The nerve turns sharply in an anterior direction to provide innervation to the anterior wall. It

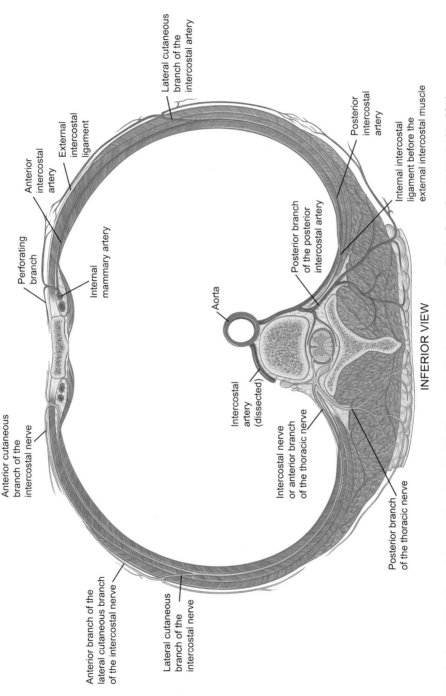

Anterior cutaneous
branch of the
intercostal nerve

Perforating
branch

Anterior
intercostal
artery

External
intercostal
ligament

Lateral cutaneous
branch of the
intercostal artery

Internal
mammary artery

Posterior
intercostal
artery

Posterior branch
of the posterior
intercostal artery

Internal intercostal
ligament before the
external intercostal muscle

Aorta

Intercostal
artery
(dissected)

Intercostal nerve
or anterior branch
of the thoracic nerve

Posterior branch
of the thoracic nerve

Anterior branch of the
lateral cutaneous branch
of the intercostal nerve

Lateral cutaneous
branch of the
intercostal nerve

INFERIOR VIEW

Fig. 5.1 Anatomy of the intercostal nerve. (From Rendina EA, Ciccone AM. The intercostal space. *Thorac Surg Clin.* 2007;17:491–501.)

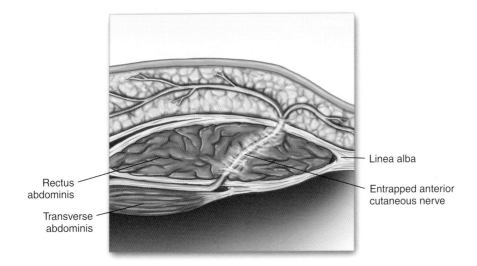

Fig. 5.2 Anatomy of the anterior cutaneous nerve. (From Waldman SD. *Atlas of Uncommon Pain Syndromes*. ed. 3. Philadelphia: Saunders; 2014.)

passes through a firm fibrous ring as it pierces the fascia, and it is at this point that the nerve is subject to entrapment. It is accompanied through the fascia by an epigastric artery and vein. Occasionally, the terminal branches of a given intercostal nerve may actually cross the midline to provide sensory innervation to the contralateral chest and abdominal wall. The 12th nerve is called the subcostal nerve and is unique because it gives off a branch to the first lumbar nerve, thus contributing to the lumbar plexus.

CLINICAL SYNDROME

Whereas most other causes of chest wall pain are musculoskeletal, the pain of intercostal neuralgia is neuropathic. As with costosternal joint pain, Tietze syndrome, and rib fractures, many patients who suffer from intercostal neuralgia seek medical attention because they believe they are having a heart attack. If the subcostal nerve is involved, gallbladder disease may be suspected. The pain of intercostal neuralgia is the result of damage to or inflammation of the intercostal nerves. The pain is constant and burning, and it may involve any of the intercostal nerves as well as the subcostal nerve of the 12th rib. The pain usually begins at the posterior axillary line and radiates anteriorly into the distribution of the affected intercostal or subcostal nerves, or both (Fig. 5.3). Deep inspiration or movement of the chest wall may slightly increase the pain of intercostal neuralgia but to a much lesser extent than with musculoskeletal causes of chest wall pain.

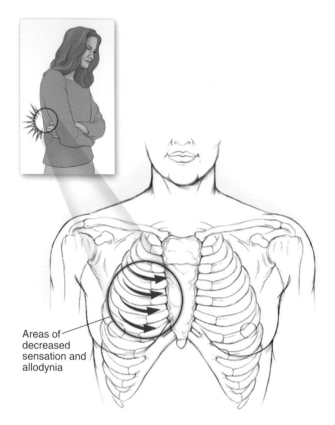

Areas of
decreased
sensation and
allodynia

Fig. 5.3 The pain of intercostal neuralgia is neuropathic rather than musculoskeletal in origin. (From Waldman S. *Atlas of Common Pain Syndromes*. ed. 4. Philadelphia: Elsevier; 2019 [Fig. 63-1].)

SIGNS AND SYMPTOMS

Physical examination generally reveals minimal findings unless the patient has a history of previous thoracic or subcostal surgery, or cutaneous evidence of herpes zoster involving the thoracic dermatomes (Fig. 5.4). Unlike patients with musculoskeletal causes of chest wall and subcostal pain, those with intercostal neuralgia do not attempt to splint or protect the affected area. Careful sensory examination of the affected dermatomes may reveal decreased sensation or allodynia. When motor involvement of the subcostal nerve is significant, the patient may complain that the abdomen bulges outward.

TESTING

Plain radiographs are indicated for all patients who present with pain thought to be emanating from the intercostal nerve to rule out occult bony disorders,

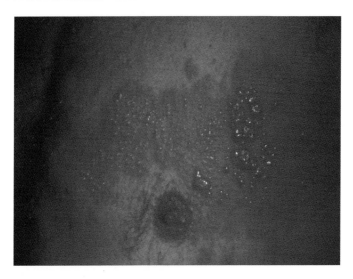

Fig. 5.4 Acute herpes zoster of the thoracic dermatome. (From Waldman S. *Atlas of Pain Management Injection Techniques*. ed. 4. St. Louis: Elsevier; 2017 [Fig. 106-1].)

including tumor (Fig. 5.5). If trauma is present, radionuclide bone scanning may be useful to exclude occult fractures of the ribs or sternum. Based on the patient's clinical presentation, additional testing may be indicated, including a complete blood count, prostate-specific antigen level, erythrocyte sedimentation rate, and antinuclear antibody testing. CT and ultrasound imaging of the ribs and thoracic contents is indicated if an occult mass is suspected (Figs. 5.6 and 5.7). Injection of the intercostal nerve with local anesthetic and steroid may serve as both a diagnostic and a therapeutic maneuver (Fig. 5.8).

DIFFERENTIAL DIAGNOSIS

As mentioned, the pain of intercostal neuralgia is often mistaken for pain of cardiac or gallbladder origin, and it leads to visits to the emergency department and unnecessary cardiac and gastrointestinal workups (Box 5.1). If trauma has occurred, intercostal neuralgia may coexist with fractured ribs or fractures of the sternum itself, which can be missed on plain radiographs and may require radionuclide bone scanning for proper identification. Tietze syndrome, which is painful enlargement of the upper costochondral cartilage associated with viral infection, may be confused with intercostal neuralgia.

Other types of neuropathic pain involving the chest wall may be confused or coexist with intercostal neuralgia. Examples of such neuropathic pain syndromes include diabetic polyneuropathies and acute herpes zoster involving the thoracic nerves. Diseases of the structures of the mediastinum and thoracic aorta

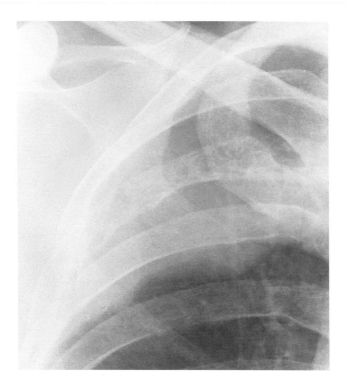

Fig. 5.5 Angiosarcoma of the ribs. An ill-defined lesion of the posterior aspect of the fourth rib is associated with a coarsened trabecular pattern and a large soft tissue mass. The osseous changes are consistent with a vascular lesion. The extent of the soft tissue involvement suggests an aggressive process. (From Resnick D. *Diagnosis of bone and joint disorders*. ed. 4. Philadelphia: Saunders; 2002:4006.)

are possible and can be difficult to diagnose (Fig. 5.9). Pathologic processes that inflame the pleura, such as pulmonary embolus, infection, and Bornholm disease, may also confuse the diagnosis and complicate treatment.

TREATMENT

Initial treatment of intercostal neuralgia includes a combination of simple analgesics and nonsteroidal antiinflammatory drugs or cyclooxygenase-2 inhibitors. If these medications do not adequately control the patient's symptoms, a tricyclic antidepressant or gabapentin should be added.

Traditionally, tricyclic antidepressants have been a mainstay in the palliation of pain caused by intercostal neuralgia. Controlled studies have demonstrated the efficacy of amitriptyline, and nortriptyline and desipramine have also proved to be clinically useful. Unfortunately, this class of drugs is associated with significant anticholinergic side effects, including dry mouth, constipation,

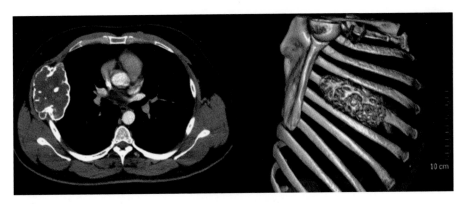

Fig. 5.6 Right chest wall mass approximately 11 cm in diameter with slightly rounded morphology, which depends on the anterior segment of the fifth rib. The profile of the mass is relatively sharp, and it has linear and anfractuous punctate calcifications inside. The rest of the content has homogenous attenuation. There was no soft tissue component, although the tumor displaces the serratus anterior muscle and pleural folds. There was no pleural effusion or mediastinal lymphadenopathy. (From Rambalde E, Parra A, Santapau A, et al. SPECT/CT with 99mTc-MDP in a patient with monostotic fibrous dysplasia of the rib. *Rev Esp Med Nucl Imag Mol.* 2013;32(2):126–127; Waldman S. *Atlas of Interventional Pain Management.* ed. 5. Philadelphia: Elsevier; 2021 [Fig. 77-2].)

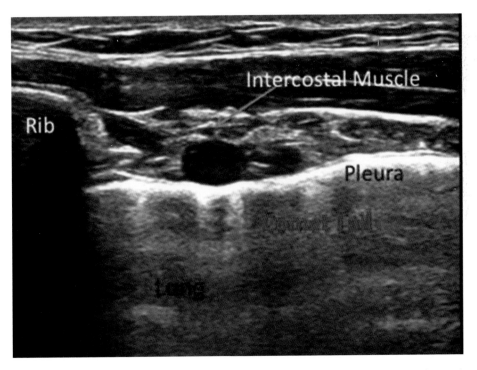

Fig. 5.7 Longitudinal ultrasound image demonstrating adjacent ribs, the intercostal muscles, and pleura with the lung beneath.

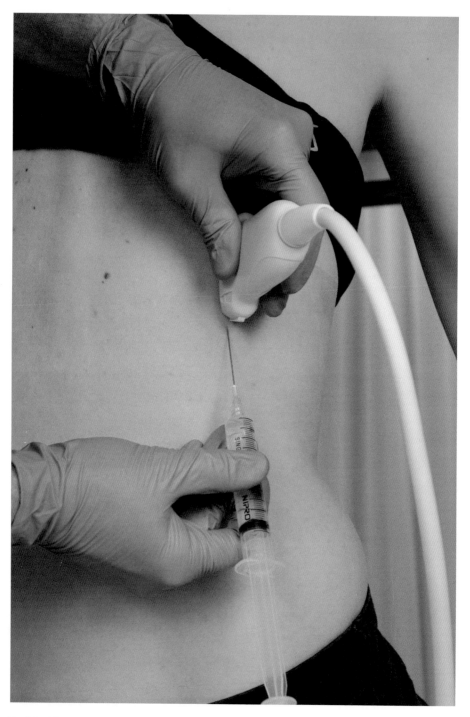

Fig. 5.8   Ultrasound-guided injection of the intercostal nerve.

BOX 5.1 ■ Differential Diagnosis of Intercostal Neuralgia

- Rib fracture
- Rib tumors (primary or metastatic)
- Chest wall contusion
- Thoracic radiculopathy
- Acute herpes zoster
- Postherpetic neuralgia
- Vertebral compression fracture
- Chostochondritis
- Tietze syndrome
- Spondylitis
- Pleurisy
- Nephrolithiasis
- Pyelonephritis
- Pulmonary embolism
- Pneumothorax
- Cholecystitis
- Esophageal disorders
- Peptic ulcer disease
- Referred cardiac pain
- Referred gastrointestinal pain
- Referred pulmonary pain

---

sedation, and urinary retention. These drugs should be used with caution in patients suffering from glaucoma, cardiac arrhythmia, and prostatism. To minimize side effects and encourage compliance, the physician should start amitriptyline or nortriptyline at a 10-mg dose at bedtime; the dose can then be titrated upward to 25 mg at bedtime, as side effects allow. Subsequently, upward titration in 25-mg increments can be carried out each week as side effects allow. Even at lower doses, patients generally report a rapid reduction in sleep disturbance and begin to experience some pain relief in 10 to 14 days. If the patient does not show any reduction in pain as the dose is being titrated upward, the addition of gabapentin alone or in combination with nerve blocks is recommended (see later). The selective serotonin reuptake inhibitors such as fluoxetine have also been used to treat the pain of intercostal neuralgia. Although these drugs are better tolerated than are the tricyclic antidepressants, they appear to be less efficacious.

If the antidepressant compounds are ineffective or contraindicated, gabapentin is a reasonable alternative. Gabapentin is started at a 300-mg dose at bedtime for 2 nights. The patient should be cautioned about potential side effects, including dizziness, sedation, confusion, and rash. The drug is then increased in 300-mg increments given in equally divided doses over 2 days as side effects allow until pain relief is obtained or a total dose of 2400 mg/day is reached. At this point, if the patient has experienced partial pain relief, blood values are measured, and the drug is carefully titrated upward using 100-mg tablets. Rarely is a

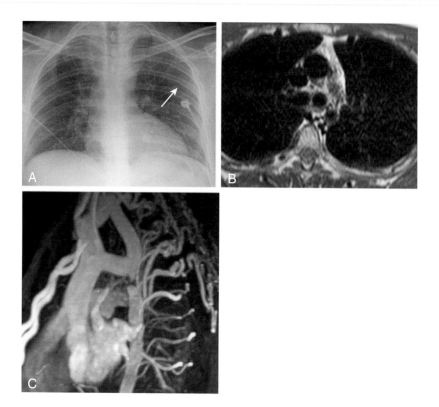

Fig. 5.9 Coarctation of the thoracic aorta with intercostal collateral vessels in a 27-year-old man evaluated for a ruptured aneurysm. (A) Frontal chest radiograph shows rib notching *(arrow)* and abnormal contour of the thoracic aorta. (B) Axial T1-weighted magnetic resonance imaging (MRI) shows large paraspinous and intercostal collateral vessels with associated flow-related signal voids. (C) Oblique sagittal maximum-intensity projected MRI shows severe coarctation of the thoracic aorta with large intercostal and internal thoracic collateral vessels. (From Lee TJ, Collins J. MR imaging evaluation of disorders of the chest wall. *Magn Reson Imaging Clin N Am.* 2008;16(2):355–379.)

dose greater than 3600 mg/day required. The local application of heat and cold or the use of an elastic rib belt may also provide symptomatic relief. For patients who do not respond to these treatment modalities, injection using local anesthetic and steroid is a reasonable next step (see Fig. 5.9).

HIGH-YIELD TAKEAWAYS

- The patient is afebrile, making an acute infectious etiology unlikely.
- The patient's symptomatology is thought to be the result of sequela of fractured ribs from a bicycle accident.

(Continued)

- Physical examination and testing should focus on the identification of pathologic processes that may mimic the clinical presentation of intercostal neuralgia.
- The patient has minimal chest wall tenderness, which suggests a neuropathic rather than musculoskeletal basis for the patient's symptoms.
- The patient's symptoms are unilateral and are localized, which is more suggestive of a local process than a systemic disease or diffuse peripheral neuropathy.
- The patient has decreased sensation in the distribution of the right 10th and 11th intercostal and subcostal nerves.
- Plain radiographs and CT scanning will provide high-yield information regarding bony abnormalities as well as abnormalities of the lung, but ultrasound imaging and MRI will be more useful in identifying soft tissue pathology.
- EMG and nerve conduction velocity testing will help delineate the location and degree of nerve compromise.

Suggested Readings

Ellis H. Anterior abdominal wall. *Anaesth Intens Care Med*. 2006;7:36–37.

Rahn DD, Phelan JN, Roshanravan SM, et al. Anterior abdominal wall nerve and vessel anatomy: clinical implications for gynecologic surgery. *Am J Obstet Gynecol*. 2010;202:234.e1–234.e5.

Vishy M. Anatomy of the anterior abdominal wall and groin. *Surgery (Oxford)*. 2009;27:251–254.

Waldman SD. Abnormalities of the rib and intercostal space. In: *Waldman's Comprehensive Atlas of Diagnostic Ultrasound of Painful Conditions*. ed. 2. Philadelphia: Wolters Kluwer; 2016:535–544.

Waldman SD. Anterior cutaneous nerve block. In: *Pain Review*. ed. 2. Philadelphia: Saunders; 2009:497–498.

Waldman SD. Fractured ribs. In: *Atlas of Common Pain Syndromes*. ed. 4. Philadelphia: Elsevier; 2019:260–264.

Waldman SD. Intercostal nerve block. In: *Atlas of Interventional Pain Management*. ed. 5. Philadelphia: Elsevier; 2021:404–412.

Waldman SD. Intercostal nerve block. In: *Pain Review*. ed. 2. Philadelphia: W.B. Saunders; 2017:454–455.

Waldman SD. The intercostal nerves. In: *Pain Review*. ed. 2. Philadelphia: W.B. Saunders; 2017:113–114.

Waldman SD. Pneumothorax, pulmonary embolism, and other abnormalities of the lung. In: *Waldman's Comprehensive Atlas of Diagnostic Ultrasound of Painful Conditions*. ed. 2. Philadelphia: Wolters Kluwer; 2016:545–560.

Waldman SD. Postmastectomy pain. In: *Atlas of Uncommon Pain Syndromes*. ed. 3. Philadelphia: W.B. Saunders; 2014:185–188.

Waldman SD. Ultrasound-guided intercostal nerve block. In: *Waldman's Comprehensive Atlas of Ultrasound-Guided Pain Management Injection Techniques*. ed. 2. Philadelphia: Wolters Kluwer; 2020:653–661.

Mark "Mo" Bandy

A 31-Year-Old Rodeo Rider With Broken Ribs After Being Thrown From a Bronco

- Learn the common causes of chest wall pain.
- Learn the common causes of fractured ribs.
- Develop an understanding of the anatomy of the ribs.
- Develop an understanding of the differential diagnosis of fractured ribs.
- Learn the clinical presentation of fractured ribs.
- Learn how to examine the lower extremity.
- Learn how to use physical examination to identify fractured ribs.
- Develop an understanding of the treatment options for fractured ribs.

Mo Bandy

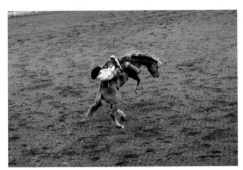

Mark "Mo" Bandy is a 31-year-old rodeo rider with the chief complaint of, "I cracked some ribs." I had been taking care of Mo for the last several years, and he was a real piece of work. Constantly nursing this injury or that, Mo was the walking textbook of musculoskeletal injuries. I had most recently treated him for a broken wrist after he was thrown from a horse. Mo had a degree in electrical engineering, but after working for a local engineering firm for less than 1 year, he just up and quit and starting riding broncos on the rodeo circuit. I had seen Mo ride, and I had to admit it was pretty impressive, but you couldn't pay me a million bucks to get on one of those crazy horses.

This time it was Mo's ribs. "Doc, you are looking a little tired. You need to get out and get some sun. Never too late to get a job as a rodeo clown." With that he started to laugh, and immediately winced in pain. "Doc, I cracked me a couple of ribs and need you to wrap me up so I can ride this weekend." I just shook my head and said, "Let me take a look."

I asked Mo how his breathing was, and he said he felt a "little winded," but it was the pain that was keeping him up at night. I asked Mo how he was sleeping, and he said, "Jack and I are sleeping just fine." "Jack?" I asked. "Doc, you know Jack." I shook my head, and said, "I don't think I've had the pleasure." Mo laughed, winced, and said, "Jack—Jack Daniels." I laughed and said that perhaps he and "Jack" should spend some time apart. "Doc, Jack is the only thing letting me get any sleep, and that is in a chair. These damn ribs are a real nuisance when it comes to my sleep." I asked Mo what he was doing for the pain, and he smiled and said, "Jack." Mo laughed, winced, and said, "Damn it, Doc! Any time I move or cough, it makes me think about a career in electrical engineering."

On physical examination, Mo was afebrile. His respirations were 18, his pulse was 78 and regular, and his blood pressure was 134/70. Mo's head, eyes, ears, nose, throat (HEENT) exam was normal. He had a lot of upper airway secretions because it hurt too much to cough, and I thought his breath sounds were somewhat decreased on the right, but it was really hard to get Mo to take a big breath because of the pain. His cardiac examination was within normal limits, but I was a little worried about his lungs. His thyroid was normal. His abdominal examination revealed no abnormal mass or organomegaly. There was no costovertebral angle

(CVA) tenderness. There was no peripheral edema. His low back examination was unremarkable. Visual inspection of Mo's right chest wall revealed a large ecchymotic area that ran from his posterior axillary line to his umbilicus. It looked like his chest had been hit with a baseball bat. The right was a little warm, but there was no obvious infection. Gentle palpation caused Mo to wince in pain. I thought I could feel a couple of free-floating rib fragments. A careful neurologic examination of the upper extremities was completely normal. Deep tendon reflexes were normal.

Key Clinical Points—What's Important and What's Not
THE HISTORY

- History of sudden onset of right chest wall pain after being thrown from a horse
- Significant bruising
- Patient notes feeling "a little winded"
- History of previous significant musculoskeletal injuries
- No fever or chills
- Significant sleep disturbance
- Pain with coughing or movement of the chest wall
- Using alcohol to treat the pain

THE PHYSICAL EXAMINATION

- Patient is afebrile
- Massive ecchymosis of the right chest wall
- Tenderness on palpation of the right chest wall
- Probable free-floating rib fragments
- Upper airway secretions secondary to inability to cough due to pain
- Questionable decreased breath sounds on the right
- No obvious infection

OTHER FINDINGS OF NOTE

- Normal HEENT examination
- Normal cardiac examination
- Normal pulmonary examination
- Normal abdominal examination
- No peripheral edema
- Normal neurologic examination

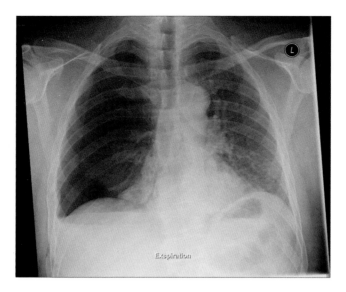

Fig. 6.1   Chest x-ray revealing right-sided fractured ribs and a pneumothorax.

What Tests Would You Like to Order?

The following tests were ordered:
- Chest x-ray
- Computed tomography (CT) of the chest

TEST RESULTS

Chest x-ray reveals fractured ribs and a pneumothorax on the right (Fig. 6.1).
CT of the right ribs reveals multiple displaced rib fractures (Fig. 6.2).

Clinical Correlation—Putting It All Together

What is the diagnosis?
- Fractured ribs

The Science Behind the Diagnosis
ANATOMY

The intercostal nerves arise from the anterior division of the thoracic paraverte-bral nerve. A typical intercostal nerve has four major branches (Fig. 6.3). The first

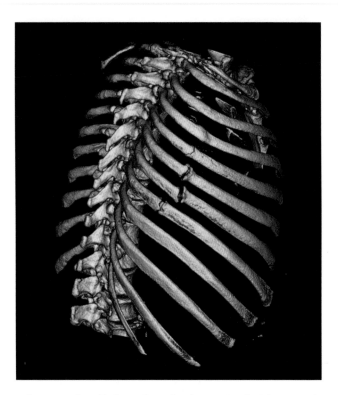

Fig. 6.2 Computed tomography with three-dimensional reconstruction demonstrating nonunion fractures on right-sided ribs following traumatic injury. (From Buehler KE, Wilshire CL, Bograd AJ, et al. Rib plating offers favorable outcomes in patients with chronic nonunion of prior rib fractures. *Ann Thorac Surg.* 2020;110(3):993–997 [Fig. 1]. ISSN 0003-4975, https://doi.org/10.1016/j.athoracsur.2020.03.075, http://www.sciencedirect.com/science/article/pii/S0003497520306159.)

branch is the unmyelinated postganglionic fibers of the gray rami communicantes, which interface with the sympathetic chain. The second branch is the posterior cutaneous branch, which innervates the muscles and skin of the paraspinal area. The third branch is the lateral cutaneous division, which arises in the anterior axillary line and provides the majority of the cutaneous innervation of the chest and abdominal wall. The fourth branch is the anterior cutaneous branch, which supplies innervation to the midline of the chest and abdominal wall (see Fig. 6.3). The anterior cutaneous branch pierces the fascia of the abdominal wall at the lateral border of the rectus abdominis muscle (Fig. 6.4). The nerve turns sharply in an anterior direction to provide innervation to the anterior wall. It passes through a firm fibrous ring as it pierces the fascia, and it is at this point that the nerve is subject to entrapment. It is accompanied through the fascia by an epigastric artery and vein. Occasionally, the terminal branches of a given intercostal nerve may actually cross the midline to provide sensory innervation to the contralateral chest and abdominal wall. The 12th nerve is called the

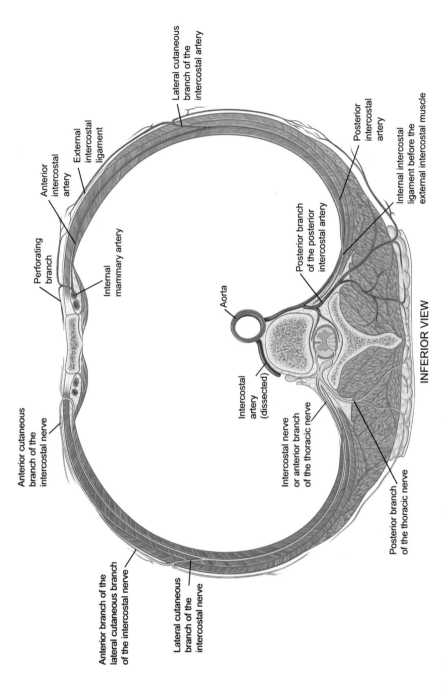

Anterior cutaneous branch of the intercostal nerve

Perforating branch

Anterior intercostal artery

External intercostal ligament

Internal mammary artery

Lateral cutaneous branch of the intercostal artery

Posterior intercostal artery

Internal intercostal ligament before the external intercostal muscle

Posterior branch of the posterior intercostal artery

Aorta

Intercostal artery (dissected)

Intercostal nerve or anterior branch of the thoracic nerve

Posterior branch of the thoracic nerve

Anterior branch of the lateral cutaneous branch of the intercostal nerve

Lateral cutaneous branch of the intercostal nerve

INFERIOR VIEW

Fig. 6.3 Anatomy of the intercostal nerve. (From Rendina EA, Ciccone AM. The intercostal space. *Thorac Surg Clin.* 2007;17:491–501.)

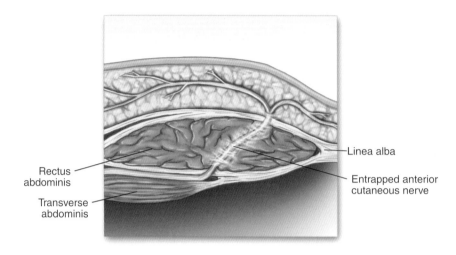

Fig. 6.4 Anatomy of the anterior cutaneous nerve. (From Waldman SD: *Atlas of Uncommon Pain Syndromes*. ed. 3. Philadelphia: Saunders; 2014.)

subcostal nerve; it is unique because it gives off a branch to the first lumbar nerve, thus contributing to the lumbar plexus.

CLINICAL SYNDROME

Fractured ribs are among the most common causes of chest wall pain. They are usually associated with trauma to the chest wall (Fig. 6.5). In osteoporotic patients or in patients with primary tumors or metastatic disease involving the ribs, fractures may occur with coughing (tussive fractures) or spontaneously.

The pain and functional disability associated with fractured ribs are largely determined by the severity of the injury (e.g., number of ribs involved), the nature of the injury (e.g., partial or complete fracture, free-floating fragments), and the amount of damage to surrounding structures, including the intercostal nerves and pleura. The pain associated with fractured ribs ranges from a dull, deep ache with partial osteoporotic fractures to severe, sharp, stabbing pain that may lead to inadequate pulmonary toilet. In the absence of significant trauma, the clinician should highly suspect the possibility of malignant lesions of the ribs (Fig. 6.6).

SIGNS AND SYMPTOMS

Rib fractures are aggravated by deep inspiration, coughing, and any movement of the chest wall. Palpation of the affected ribs may elicit pain and

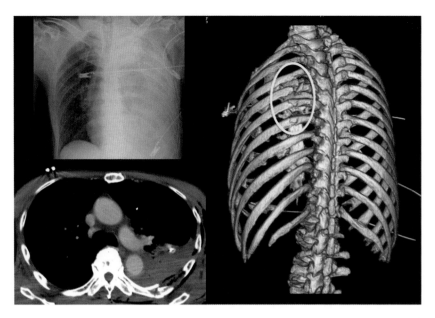

Fig. 6.5 Chest radiography and computed tomography (CT) performed in a supine position on admission in the local hospital. Chest radiography and CT showed multiple left rib fractures and massive hemothorax *(circle)*. The fractured fourth to seventh ribs are shown on three-dimensional chest CT scan. (From Goda Y, Shoji T, Date N, et al. Hemothorax resulting from an initially masked aortic perforation caused by penetration of the sharp edge of a fractured rib: a case report. *Int J Surg Case Rep.* 2020;68:18−21 [Fig. 1]. ISSN 2210-2612, https://doi.org/10.1016/j.ijscr.2020.02.023, http://www.sciencedirect.com/science/article/pii/S2210261220300973.)

reflex spasm of the musculature of the chest wall. Ecchymosis overlying the fractures may be present. The clinician should be aware of the possibility of pneumothorax or hemopneumothorax (see Fig. 6.1). Fracture of the first rib may result in trauma to the cervical sympathetic ganglia and produce a Horner syndrome (Fig. 6.7). Damage to the intercostal nerves may produce severe pain and result in reflex splinting of the chest wall that further compromises the patient's pulmonary status. Failure to treat this pain and splinting aggressively may result in a negative cycle of hypoventilation, atelectasis, and (ultimately) pneumonia.

TESTING

Plain radiographs or CT scans of the ribs and chest are indicated for all patients who present with pain from fractured ribs to rule out occult fractures and other bony disorders, including tumor, as well as pneumothorax and hemopneumothorax (see Figs. 6.1 and 6.2). If trauma is present, radionuclide bone scanning

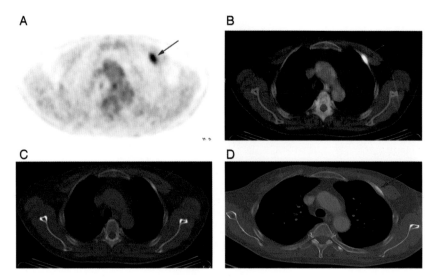

Fig. 6.6 18F-fluorodeoxyglucose (FDG) positron emission tomography/computed tomography (PET/CT) scan of a 68-year-old male for restaging of non−small cell lung cancer after chemotherapy and radiation therapy. Discrete focal FDG uptake (SUVmax 5.2) was present in left second rib *(arrows)* on (A) PET and (B) PET/CT fusion axial images. Osteoblastic lesion was noted on (C) bone window setting CT image. After 9 months, osteoblastic lesion *(arrow)* showed progression even after chemotherapy on (D) chest CT images, and it was considered to be bony metastatic disease. (From Choi HS, Yoo IR, Park HL, et al. Role of 18F-FDG PET/CT in differentiation of a benign lesion and metastasis on the ribs of cancer patients. *Clin Imag.* 2014;38(2):109−114 [Fig. 3]. ISSN 0899-7071, https://doi.org/10.1016/j.clinimag. 2013.11.011, http://www.sciencedirect.com/science/article/pii/S0899707113003185.)

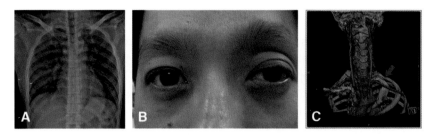

Fig. 6.7 (A) Chest radiography showing right chest contusion with fractures of the right second, third, and fourth ribs. (B) The clinical picture with left eye ptosis. (C) Three-dimensional reconstructed computed tomographic angiography reveals a rare transverse fracture in the left first rib *(arrow)* without left carotid artery dissection. (From Lin Y-C, Chuang M-T, Hsu C-H, Tailor A-R A, Lee J-S. First rib fracture resulting in Horner's syndrome. *J Emerg Med.* 2015;49(6):868−870.)

may be useful to exclude occult fractures of the ribs or sternum (see Fig. 6.6). If no trauma is present, bone density testing to rule out osteoporosis is appropriate, as are serum protein electrophoresis and testing for hyperparathyroidism. Based on the patient's clinical presentation, additional testing may be warranted,

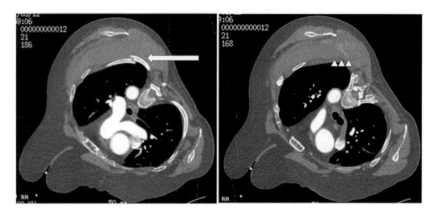

Fig. 6.8 Computed tomography taken on day 26 with the patient in right lateral decubitus position because of severe left back pain. This scan reveals posterior fracture of the left sixth rib *(arrow)* and an enlargement of the chest wall hematoma with extravasation *(arrowhead)*. (From Sato N, Sekiguchi H, Hirose Y, Yoshida S. Delayed chest wall hematoma caused by progressive displacement of rib fractures after blunt trauma. *Trauma Case Rep*. 2016;4:1—4.)

including a complete blood count, prostate-specific antigen level, erythrocyte sedimentation rate, and antinuclear antibody testing. CT and magnetic resonance imaging (MRI) of the thoracic contents, soft tissues, and adjacent organs are indicated if an occult mass or significant trauma to the thoracic contents is suspected (Fig. 6.8). Electrocardiography is recommended for all patients with traumatic sternal fractures or significant anterior chest wall trauma to exclude cardiac contusion. The injection technique described later should be used early to avoid pulmonary complications.

DIFFERENTIAL DIAGNOSIS

In the trauma setting, diagnosis of fractured ribs is usually straightforward. In the setting of spontaneous rib fracture secondary to cough, osteoporosis, or metastatic disease, diagnosis may be less clear-cut, and medical imaging is indicated (Fig. 6.9). In this case, the pain of occult rib fracture is often mistaken for pain of cardiac or gallbladder origin, and it leads to visits to the emergency department and unnecessary cardiac and gastrointestinal workups. Tietze syndrome, which is painful enlargement of the upper costochondral cartilage associated with viral infection, may be confused with fractured ribs, especially if the patient has been coughing.

TREATMENT

Initial treatment of rib fracture pain includes a combination of simple analgesics and nonsteroidal antiinflammatory drugs or cyclooxygenase-2 inhibitors.

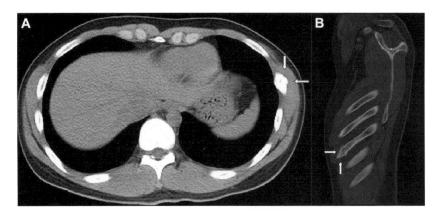

Fig. 6.9 (A) Axial view. (B) Saggital view. Chest computed tomography scan shows a cough-induced (tussive) fracture of the left seventh rib with callus formation *(white arrows)*. (From Yeh C-F, Su S-C. Cough-induced rib fracture in a young healthy man. *J Formosan Med Assoc.* 2012;111(3):179–180 [Fig. 1]. ISSN 0929-6646, https://doi.org/10.1016/j.jfma.2011.07.020, http://www.sciencedirect.com/science/article/pii/S0929664612001210.)

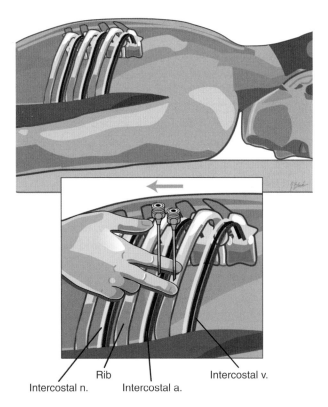

Fig. 6.10 Injection technique for fractured ribs. (From Waldman SD. *Atlas of Interventional Pain Management.* ed. 4. Philadelphia: Saunders; 2015.)

If these medications do not adequately control the patient's symptoms, short-acting opioid analgesics such as hydrocodone are a reasonable next step. Because opioid analgesics have the potential to suppress the cough reflex and respiration, the patient must be closely monitored and instructed in adequate pulmonary toilet techniques. Transdermal lidocaine patches may also be used in conjunction with pharmacologic management of rib fracture pain.

The local application of heat and cold or the use of an elastic rib belt may also provide symptomatic relief. For patients who do not respond to these treatment modalities, injection using local anesthetic and steroid should be implemented to avoid pulmonary complications (Fig. 6.10).

HIGH-YIELD TAKEAWAYS

- The patient is afebrile, making an acute infectious etiology unlikely.
- The patient's symptomatology is thought to be the result of acute trauma from being thrown from a horse.
- Physical examination and testing should focus on the identification of diseases that mimic fractured ribs.
- The patient exhibits physical examination findings that are suggestive of fractured ribs, which is a radiographic diagnosis.
- The patient's symptoms are unilateral, suggestive of a local process rather than a systemic inflammatory process.
- Plain radiographs provide high-yield information regarding the bony contents of the joint and the presence of fractured ribs, but ultrasound imaging and MRI may be more useful in identifying soft tissue pathology that is responsible for compromise of the contents of the ribs.
- CT scanning and radionucleotide imaging may help identify occult fractures and tumors.

Suggested Readings

Marco CA, Sorensen D, Hardman C, et al. Risk factors for pneumonia following rib fractures. *Am J Emerg Med*. 2020;38(3):610–612.

Waldman SD. Abnormalities of the rib and intercostal space. In: *Waldman's Comprehensive Atlas of Diagnostic Ultrasound of Painful Conditions*. ed. 2. Philadelphia: Wolters Kluwer; 2016:535–544.

Waldman SD. Fractured ribs. In: *Atlas of Common Pain Syndromes*. ed. 4. Philadelphia: Elsevier; 2017:260–264.

Waldman SD. Intercostal nerve block. In: *Atlas of Interventional Pain Management*. ed. 5. Philadelphia: Elsevier; 2021:404–412.

Waldman SD. Intercostal nerve block. In: *Pain Review*. ed. 2. Philadelphia: W.B. Saunders; 2017:454–455.

Waldman SD. The intercostal nerves. In: *Pain Review*. ed. 2. Philadelphia: W.B. Saunders; 2017:113–114.

Waldman SD. Pneumothorax, pulmonary embolism, and other abnormalities of the lung. In: *Waldman's Comprehensive Atlas of Diagnostic Ultrasound of Painful Conditions*. ed. 2. Philadelphia: Wolters Kluwer; 2016:545–560.

Waldman SD. Ultrasound-guided intercostal nerve block. In: *Waldman's Comprehensive Atlas of Ultrasound-Guided Pain Management Injection Techniques*. ed. 2. Philadelphia: Wolters Kluwer; 2020:653–661.

Laura McIlhenny

A 26-Year-Old Cosmetic Salesperson With Severe Knifelike Pain and a Clicking Sensation in the Lower Ribs Following a Seatbelt Injury

LEARNING OBJECTIVES

- Learn the common causes of chest wall pain.
- Develop an understanding of the innervation of the chest wall and pelvis.
- Develop an understanding of the anatomy of the chest wall.
- Develop an understanding of the causes of slipping rib syndrome.
- Learn the clinical presentation of slipping rib syndrome.
- Learn how to use physical examination to identify slipping rib syndrome.
- Develop an understanding of the treatment options for slipping rib syndrome.
- Learn the appropriate testing options to help diagnose slipping rib syndrome.
- Learn to identify red flags in patients who present with chest wall pain.
- Develop an understanding of the role in interventional pain management in the treatment of slipping rib syndrome.

Laura McIlhenny

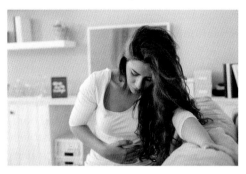

Laura McIlhenny is a 26-year-old cosmetic salesperson with the chief complaint of, "I feel like somebody is stabbing me in the ribs with a knife." Laura went on to say that she was involved in a motor vehicle accident. A distracted driver slammed into the back of her car when she was sitting at a stoplight. The impact threw her forward against her seatbelt. She was shaken up, but her car was driveable, and she went on to work. Her lower ribs on the right were sore, but she thought she would be fine. That evening, when walking out to the parking lot after work, Laura stated that she felt a sudden, sharp, stabbing pain in her right lower ribs. "At first, I thought I had been stabbed, that someone was trying to mug me. You can't believe how bad the pain was. It doubled me over. It lasted for a minute or so and then went away as quickly as it came. The odd thing was, when I went to stand up, I felt like my ribs popped back into place, kind of a clicking sensation. It's hard to describe, but it was very weird and rather nauseating." Laura went on to say, "Doctor, do you think I could be pregnant or have some kind of cancer? I did a home pregnancy test, but it could have been too soon because I just had my period." Laura said that she was really having a hard time getting the pain better in spite of trying a massage and aromatherapy. Her friend at work gave her a lidocaine patch, which seemed to help a bit. She said she took some pain pills that were left over from when she had her wisdom teeth pulled. They helped a little, but they made her loopy.

I asked Laura if she ever had anything like this happen before, and she shook her head no. She also denied any current urinary or gynecologic symptoms, hematuria, or fever or chills. She also denied a history of kidney stones. Her last menstrual period was about 5 days ago. Laura was using oral contraceptives, but she volunteered that she was fearful of having sex because she didn't want to trigger the pain. I asked her to rate her pain on a 1 to 10 scale, with 10 being the worst pain she had ever had, and she said the pain was an 11 when it hit and a 1 after it went away. "Doctor, this pain is really scaring me. I'm scared to move for fear of triggering it. The pain is interfering with just about everything. I am afraid to bend over to tie my shoes or shave my legs. I have a hard time getting dressed, no exercise, no sex—it's ruining everything. I just really need to get my life back."

I asked Laura to point with one finger to show me where it hurts the most. She pointed to the area over her right lower ribs, and said, "Doctor, the pain is right here. This is where the clicking comes from. This is the spot, right here on top of the ribs."

On physical examination, Laura was afebrile. Her respirations were 16. Her pulse was 72 and regular. Her blood pressure was normal at 118/68. Her head, eyes, ears, nose, throat (HEENT) exam was normal, as was her thyroid examination. Her cardiopulmonary examination was negative. Her abdominal examination revealed no abnormal mass or organomegaly. Examination over the right costochondral cartilage revealed some tenderness to deep palpation. Costochondral instability of the eighth rib on the right was noted, and a clicking sensation was noted with downward pressure on the costochondral cartilage. No mass or abdominal wall hernia was identified. Visual inspection of the painful area revealed no ecchymosis or evidence of infection. There was no costovertebral angle (CVA) tenderness. There was no peripheral edema. Her low back examination was unremarkable. When I asked Laura to stand up and walk, I noticed that she got up very carefully and walked with her thoracic spine flexed to splint the affected costochondral cartilage. Her lower extremity neurologic examination was completely normal. The hooking maneuver test for slipping rib syndrome was markedly positive on the right (Fig. 7.1). I said, "Laura, I think I know what's going on, and I have a pretty good idea of how to get you better." Laura gave me a tentative smile and said, "I certainly hope so. This has been really upsetting."

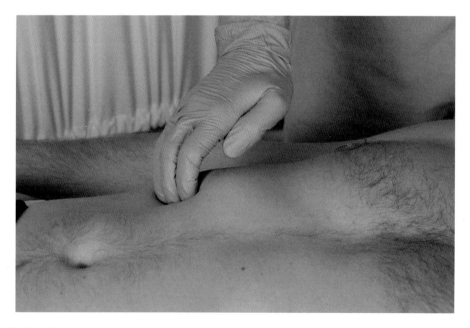

Fig. 7.1   The hooking maneuver test for slipping rib syndrome.

Key Clinical Points—What's Important and What's Not

THE HISTORY

- History of recent onset of right chest wall pain following a seatbelt injury
- No history of gynecologic or urinary tract symptoms related to the pain
- No history of kidney stones
- No history of hematuria
- Character of pain is sharp, stabbing, and knifelike
- Clicking sensation associated with the pain
- Difficulty in carrying out activities of daily living
- Pain localized to the origin of the right chest wall
- No fever or chills

THE PHYSICAL EXAMINATION

- Patient is afebrile
- Normal visual inspection of the right chest wall with no ecchymosis noted
- Palpation of the right lower chest wall elicited only mild pain
- Costochondral instability of the eighth costochondral cartilage
- Patient walks with flexed thoracic spine in an attempt to splint the affected costochondral cartilage
- Hooking maneuver test for slipping rib syndrome markedly positive on the right
- No abnormal mass or abdominal wall hernia identified

OTHER FINDINGS OF NOTE

- Normal blood pressure
- Normal HEENT examination
- Normal cardiopulmonary examination
- Normal abdominal examination
- No peripheral edema
- No CVA tenderness

What Tests Would You Like to Order?

The following tests were ordered:
- X-ray of right ribs
- Chest x-ray
- Dynamic ultrasound imaging of the painful costochondral cartilage
- Pregnancy test
- Urinalysis

TEST RESULTS

Plain radiograph of the ribs is reported as normal.

Chest x-ray is reported as normal.

Dynamic ultrasound imaging of the lower costochondral cartilage on the right is reported as positive with subluxation of the eighth costochondral cartilage (Fig. 7.2).

Pregnancy test is negative.

Clinical Correlation—Putting It All Together

What is the diagnosis?
- Slipping rib syndrome

The Science Behind the Diagnosis

ANATOMY OF THE CHEST WALL

The cartilage of the true ribs articulates with the sternum via the costosternal joints (Fig. 7.3). The cartilage of the first rib articulates directly with the manubrium of the sternum and is a synarthrodial joint that allows a limited gliding movement. The cartilage of the second through sixth ribs articulates with the body of the sternum via true arthrodial joints. These joints are surrounded by a thin articular capsule. The costosternal joints are strengthened by ligaments. The eighth, ninth, and tenth ribs attach to the costal cartilage of the rib directly above. The cartilages of the 11th and 12th ribs are called floating ribs because they end in the abdominal musculature (see Fig. 7.3). The pleural space and peritoneal cavity may be entered when performing the following injection technique if the needle is placed too deeply and laterally, and pneumothorax or damage to the abdominal viscera may result.

CLINICAL SYNDROME

Encountered more frequently in clinical practice since the increased use of across-the-chest seatbelts and airbags, slipping rib syndrome is often misdiagnosed, leading to prolonged suffering and excessive testing for intraabdominal and intrathoracic pathologic conditions. Slipping rib syndrome is a constellation of symptoms consisting of severe knifelike pain emanating from the lower costal cartilages associated with hypermobility of the anterior end of the lower costal cartilages. The 10th rib is most commonly involved, but the eighth and ninth ribs also can be affected. This syndrome is also known as the rib-tip syndrome (Box 7.1). Slipping rib syndrome is almost always associated with trauma to the

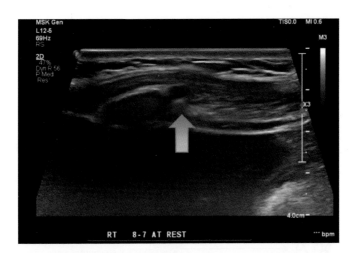

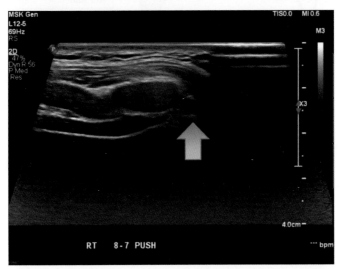

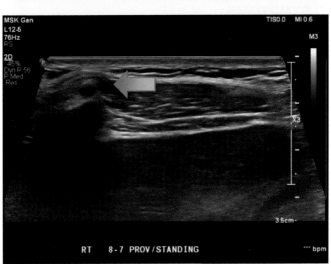

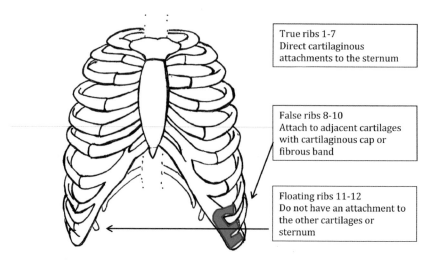

True ribs 1-7
Direct cartilaginous
attachments to the sternum

False ribs 8-10
Attach to adjacent cartilages
with cartilaginous cap or
fibrous band

Floating ribs 11-12
Do not have an attachment to
the other cartilages or
sternum

Fig. 7.3 Anatomy of the ribs and associated cartilage. Note that ribs 8 to 10 are also called the false or floating ribs because they do not directly attach to the sternum. These are the main ribs at risk for slipping rib syndrome. (From McMahon LE. Slipping rib syndrome: a review of evaluation, diagnosis and treatment. *Sem Pediatr Surg.* 2018;27(3):183–188 [Fig. 1]. ISSN 1055-8586, https://doi.org/10.1053/j.sempedsurg. 2018.05.009, http://www.sciencedirect.com/science/article/pii/S1055858618300349.)

costal cartilage of the lower ribs. These cartilages are often traumatized during acceleration-deceleration injuries and blunt trauma to the chest. With severe trauma, the cartilage may sublux or dislocate from the ribs. Patients with slipping rib syndrome may report a clicking sensation with movement of the affected ribs and associated cartilage.

SIGNS AND SYMPTOMS

On physical examination, the patient vigorously attempts to splint the affected costal cartilage joints by keeping the thoracolumbar spine slightly flexed (Fig. 7.4). Pain is reproduced with pressure on the affected costal cartilage. Patients with slipping rib syndrome exhibit a positive hooking maneuver test. The hooking maneuver test is performed by having the patient lie in the supine position with the abdominal muscles relaxed while the clinician hooks

◀ **Fig. 7.2** Dynamic ultrasound demonstrating slipping rib 8 at rest, with a push on the lower costal cartilage and with a provocative hooking maneuver, demonstrating abnormal movement of the cartilage *(blue arrows)*. (From McMahon LE. Slipping rib syndrome: a review of evaluation, diagnosis and treatment. *Sem Pediatr Surg.* 2018;27(3):183–188 [Fig. 8]. ISSN 1055-8586, https://doi.org/10.1053/j. sempedsurg.2018.05.009, http://www.sciencedirect.com/science/article/pii/S1055858618300349.)

BOX 7.1 ■ Other Names for Slipping Rib Syndrome

- Rib tip syndrome
- Floating rib syndrome
- Painful gliding rib syndrome
- Clicking rib syndrome
- Cyriax syndrome
- Painful rib syndrome
- Slipping rib cartilage syndrome
- Twelfth rib syndrome
- Subluxing rib syndrome

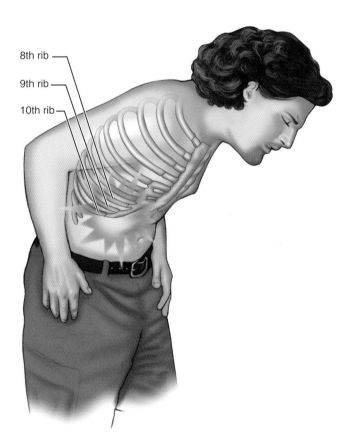

8th rib

9th rib

10th rib

Fig. 7.4 Patients with slipping rib syndrome will often flex the thoracic spine in an attempt to splint the affected costochondral cartilage. (From Waldman S. *Atlas of Uncommon Pain Syndromes*. ed. 4. Philadelphia: Elsevier; 2020 [Fig. 72-1].)

the fingers under the lower rib cage and pulls gently outward. Pain and a clicking or snapping sensation of the affected ribs and cartilage indicate a positive test.

TESTING

Plain radiographs are indicated in all patients who present with pain thought to be emanating from the lower costal cartilage and ribs to rule out occult bony pathologic processes, including rib fracture and tumor (Fig. 7.5). Based on the patient's clinical presentation, additional tests (complete blood cell count, prostate-specific antigen level, erythrocyte sedimentation rate, and antinuclear antibody testing) may be indicated. Dynamic ultrasound imaging can be useful in identifying costochondral instability associated with slipping rib syndrome (see Fig. 7.2). Magnetic resonance imaging (MRI) and computed tomography

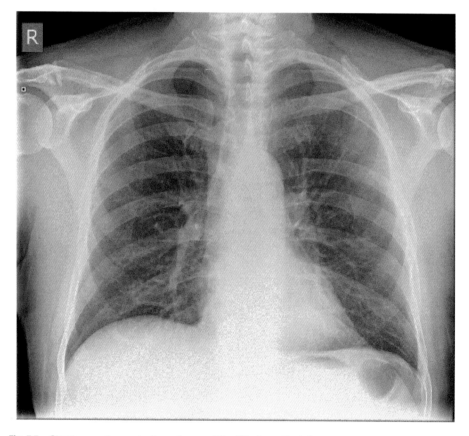

Fig. 7.5 Chest x-ray demonstrating a tumor of the fifth rib on the left.

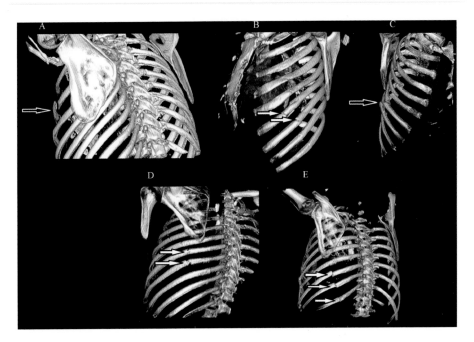

Fig. 7.6 Computed tomography three-dimensional reconstructions of the different patterns of rib fractures *(arrows):* (A) Upper rib (rib 3). (B) Anterior middle ribs. (C) Lateral middle ribs. (D) Posterior middle ribs. (E) Lower ribs. (From Pines G, Gotler Y, Lazar LO, et al. Clinical significance of rib fractures' anatomical patterns. *Injury.* 2020;51(8):1812−1816 [Fig. 2]. ISSN 0020-1383, https://doi.org/10.1016/j. injury.2020.05.023, http://www.sciencedirect.com/science/article/pii/S0020138320304290.)

(CT) scanning of the affected ribs and cartilage are indicated if joint instability, fracture, or occult mass is suspected (Fig. 7.6). The injection of the affected costal cartilage with local anesthetic and steroid may serve as a diagnostic and therapeutic maneuver (Fig. 7.7).

DIFFERENTIAL DIAGNOSIS

As mentioned earlier, the pain of slipping rib syndrome is often mistaken for pain of cardiac or gallbladder origin and can lead to visits to the emergency department and unnecessary cardiac and gastrointestinal workups. If trauma has occurred, slipping rib syndrome may coexist with rib fractures or fractures of the sternum, which can be missed on plain radiographs and may require radionuclide bone scanning for proper identification. Tietze syndrome, which is painful enlargement of the upper costochondral cartilage associated with viral infections, can be confused with slipping rib syndrome, as can devil's grip, which is a pleura-based pain syndrome of infectious origin.

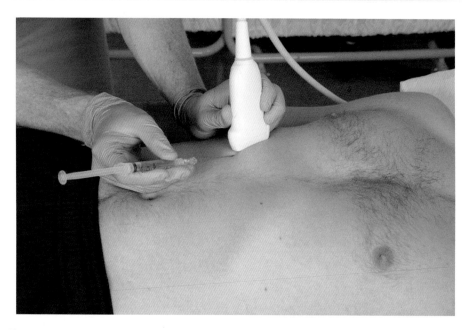

Fig. 7.7   Ultrasound-guided injection for slipping rib syndrome.

Neuropathic pain involving the chest wall also may be confused or coexist with slipping rib syndrome. Examples of such neuropathic pain include diabetic polyneuropathies and acute herpes zoster involving the thoracic nerves. The possibility of diseases of the structures of the mediastinum is ever present, and these diseases sometimes can be difficult to diagnose. Pathologic processes that inflame the pleura, such as pulmonary embolus, infection, and tumor, also should be considered.

TREATMENT

Initial treatment of the pain and functional disability associated with slipping rib syndrome should include a combination of nonsteroidal antiinflammatory drugs or cyclooxygenase-2 inhibitors and physical therapy. The local application of heat and cold may be beneficial. The repetitive movements that incite the syndrome should be avoided. For patients who do not respond to these treatment modalities, injection of the affected costochondral cartilages with a local anesthetic and steroid may be a reasonable next step (see Fig. 7.7). If conservative measures are ineffective, excision of the offending cartilage may be required (Fig. 7.8).

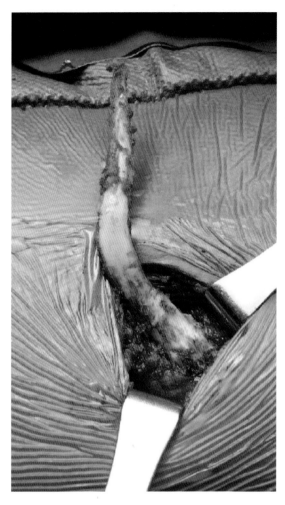

Fig. 7.8 Left-sided slipping rib excision. A small incision can be made and tissues mobilized to remove the slipping cartilage and rib. (From McMahon LE. Slipping rib syndrome: a review of evaluation, diagnosis and treatment. *Sem Pediatr Surg*. 2018;27(3):183–188. ISSN 1055-8586, https://doi.org/10.1053/j.sempedsurg.2018.05.009, http://www.sciencedirect.com/science/article/pii/S1055858618300349.)

HIGH-YIELD TAKEAWAYS

- The patient's symptomatology began after a seatbelt injury.
- The patient's pain is localized to the costochondral junction of the eighth, ninth, and tenth ribs.
- The patient has a positive hooking maneuver test, which is highly suggestive of slipping rib syndrome.

(Continued)

- The patient is afebrile, making an acute infectious etiology (e.g., urosepsis) unlikely.
- The patient's urinalysis is normal, which makes nephrolithiasis unlikely.

Suggested Readings

Fares MY, Dimassi Z, Baydoun H, et al. Slipping rib syndrome: solving the mystery of the shooting pain. *Am J Med Sci.* 2019;357(2):168–173.

Hansen AJ, Toker A, Hayanga J, et al. Minimally invasive repair of adult slipped rib syndrome without costal cartilage excision. *Ann Thorac Surg.* 2020;110(3):1030–1035.

McMahon LE. Slipping rib syndrome: a review of evaluation, diagnosis and treatment. *Sem Pediatr Surg.* 2018;27(3):183–188.

Turcios NL. Slipping rib syndrome: an elusive diagnosis. *Paediatr Resp Rev.* 2017;22:44–46.

van Delft EAK, van Pul KM, Bloemers FW. The slipping rib syndrome: a case report. *Int J Surg Case Rep.* 2016;23:23–24.

Waldman SD. Slipping rib syndrome. In: *Waldman's Comprehensive Atlas of Diagnostic Ultrasound of Painful Conditions.* ed. 2. Philadelphia: Wolters Kluwer; 2016:561–565.

Waldman SD. Ultrasound-guided injection technique for slipping rib syndrome. In: *Waldman's Comprehensive Atlas of Ultrasound-Guided Pain Management Injection Techniques.* ed. 2. Philadelphia: Wolters Kluwer; 2020:676–684.

Amy Cleaves

A 30-Year-Old Female With Shooting Chest Pain

LEARNING OBJECTIVES

- Learn the common causes of chest pain.
- Develop an understanding of the etiology of precordial catch syndrome.
- Learn the clinical presentation of precordial catch syndrome.
- Learn how to use physical examination to rule out pathology and other chest pain syndromes that may mimic precordial catch syndrome.
- Develop an understanding of the treatment options for precordial catch syndrome.
- Learn the appropriate testing options to help diagnose precordial catch syndrome.
- Learn to identify red flags in patients who present with chest pain.

Amy Cleaves

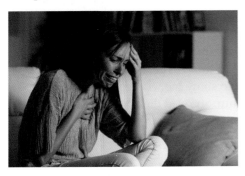

Amy Cleaves is a 30-year-old Web designer with the chief complaint of, "I think I am having a heart attack!" Amy started to speak again, and broke out in tears. "Doctor, I am really scared! Who will take care of my kids? How did this happen? What am I going to do?" I did what I could to calm Amy and promised her that together, we would figure this out. I asked Amy to describe her symptoms. Amy said, "Out of nowhere, I get this sharp pain on the left side of my breastbone just over my heart. It really hurts! It's there and it goes away as quickly as it comes. It really scares me each time it happens!" I asked, "So, Amy, what does the pain feel like, an ache, a stab, an electric shock?" She said, "Doctor, the pain is like a sharp jab that goes right into my heart. One second I am fine, and the next second it hits, it lasts for a second or two, and then it is gone." "Amy, does it hurt between attacks?" She shook her head and said maybe just a little, but she wondered if that pain was more from her rubbing the painful spot and making it sore rather than coming from her heart. "Amy, what are you doing when the pain comes on?" "That's the crazy thing, I can be sitting with the kids watching *Sesame Street* and it hits. The kids can tell it's happening. I try to hide it, but it just hurts so bad." At that, Amy started crying again. I again tried to calm her down and then asked if the pain went anywhere, like down her arm, into her jaw, or somewhere else, and she shook her head no. I continued, "Any sweating, palpations, fever, chills, shortness of breath, cough, leg pain, anything else I need to know about?" Amy responded, "Not really, Doctor, but I read on the Internet that heart attacks in women are different than heart attacks in men." "That's true," I said, "and we need to take this very seriously. The first step is to check out your heart and then figure out what the exact cause of this pain is."

I asked Amy to rate her chest pain on a 1 to 10 scale, with 10 being the worst pain she had ever had, and she said, "This pain is a 20. Doc, this is worse than anything I have ever had. Worse than when my son Jimmie slammed my hand in the car door, worse than having a baby. It's killing me! I just can't go on like this!"

I asked Amy if she had any fever or chills since her pain begin, and she shook her head no. She admitted that she quit taking her birth control pills because of the chest pain, as she had read on the Internet that birth control pills cause blood clots. "But honestly, Doctor, with this chest pain, sex is out of the question. I don't want to have a heart attack and drop dead while I'm having sex with my partner."

I asked Amy if she ever had anything like this before, and she shook her head no. I asked what she was doing to manage the pain, and she reported, "nothing really works." She tried a heating pad, but it really didn't seem to help. She went on to say, "Doctor, I have nobody. I don't know what will happen to my kids if I have a heart attack. What can I do?" I reassured her that together, we would get this sorted out, and I would do everything I could to get her better.

I asked Amy to point with one finger to show me where it hurt the most. She pointed to an area to the left of her sternum. She said that she kept looking in the mirror expecting to see something there. "Doc, you can't see anything. There is nothing there. It's down deep inside. I am afraid it's something really bad." I again reassured Amy that we would figure out what was going on and that I would do everything I could to get her better. She gave me a weak smile and said that she hoped so because she was really worn out with the whole thing. "Amy, since this pain has been so hard on you, I have a couple of questions, and I want you to really think before answering because the answers are very important." She said, "Okay, Doctor, I will do my best." I said that I knew she would. I then asked her, "Amy, have you ever felt like life just isn't worth living?" She seemed shocked and then answered, "Doctor, if you are asking me if this pain makes me want to kill myself, the answer is absolutely not. That is a sin, and besides, I have everything to live for, my kids, my partner, my job. I love them all. I would never even think about such a horrible thing. My kids come first, before everyone and everything. They are such good kids." I responded, "Okay, that's good, but I want you to know that you can tell me anything, no judgments, no criticism. I'm always here to help." She smiled and said that she really appreciated my concern, that she always knew that she could count on me. "So, next question. Do you feel like you have an excess of worry or stress? You mentioned that you have been really scared and worried about the pain." Amy thought for a moment and admitted that she had been pretty stressed out, but quickly went on to say, "Doctor, I am not imagining this or making it up! The pain is not in my head. It's coming from my heart." I reassured her, "Okay, Amy, that's good to know. One last question. Are you being hurt or abused, or have you been hurt or abused in a past relationship or by a stranger or loved one?" Amy shook her head no, and said, "Absolutely not. I have a wonderful partner who is loving and would never hurt me. My kids' father was a kind man, too. That relationship just wasn't meant to be. He drifted out of my life when I got pregnant with our youngest, and I have no idea where he is now. With my current partner, I feel very blessed." I again reassured her, "Amy, this is a place where you can always talk. You can always come for help." She nodded yes, and said she knew that. She said she appreciated my concern and it meant so much to her. I felt pretty good about that!

On physical examination, Amy was afebrile. Her respirations were 16. Her pulse was 72 and regular. Her blood pressure was normal at 118/74. Her head, eyes, ears, nose, throat (HEENT) exam was normal, as was her thyroid examination. Her cardiopulmonary examination was completely negative. Specifically, her lungs were clear, and there was no mitral valve click suggestive of mitral valve prolapse or cardiac arrythmia. She had mild tenderness over the left costosternal area, but there was no obvious mass, costochondritis, or swelling of the joints suggestive of Tietze syndrome. There were no cutaneous lesions suggestive of herpes zoster or evidence of previous trauma. There was no evidence of infection. Her breast examination was normal. Her abdominal examination revealed no abnormal mass or organomegaly. There was no costovertebral angle (CVA) tenderness. There was no peripheral edema or findings suggestive of thrombophlebitis. Her low back examination was unremarkable. Her lower extremity neurologic examination was completely normal.

I told Amy that I had good news. "I didn't find anything bad on your examination. And more good news. There's nothing to make me believe your pain is from the heart, but we aren't going to take any chances." I had a good idea about what was wrong and how to fix it. For the first time, Amy smiled and said, "Thank you, Doctor. I know I can always count on you."

Key Clinical Points—What's Important and What's Not

THE HISTORY

- History of sharp, paroxysmal chest pain without a history of antecedent trauma
- Patient's strong belief that she was having a heart attack
- No classic signs of angina
- Admits to increased anxiety related to the pain
- Pain is localized to the left parasternal area
- No fever or chills
- Denies suicidal ideation
- Denies domestic violence or abuse

THE PHYSICAL EXAMINATION

- Patient is afebrile
- Normal visual inspection of the chest wall
- Normal cardiac examination
- No mitral valve click on auscultation
- No cardiac arrythmia noted
- Normal pulmonary and abdominal exam
- No evidence of thrombophlebitis
- No evidence of Tietze syndrome

- No evidence of costochondritis
- Normal breast examination

OTHER FINDINGS OF NOTE

- Normal blood pressure
- Normal HEENT examination
- No peripheral edema
- No chest mass or evidence of infection
- No CVA tenderness

 What Tests Would You Like to Order?

The following tests were ordered:
- Chest x-ray
- Electrocardiogram (ECG)
- Cardiac stress echocardiography test

TEST RESULTS

Chest x-ray is reported as normal.

ECG is completely within normal limits with no evidence of arrythmia or cardiac ischemia.

The cardiac stress test is reported as normal with no evidence of left ventricular wall dysfunction or ischemia on ECG. The ejection fraction is reported as 72%.

 Clinical Correlation—Putting It All Together

What is the diagnosis?
- Precordial catch syndrome

The Science Behind the Diagnosis
ANATOMY

The cartilage of the true ribs articulates with the sternum via the costosternal joints (Fig. 8.1). The cartilage of the first rib articulates directly with the manubrium of the sternum and is a synarthrodial joint that allows a limited gliding movement. The cartilage of the second through sixth ribs articulates with the body of the sternum via true arthrodial joints. These joints are surrounded by a thin articular capsule. The costosternal joints are strengthened by ligaments.

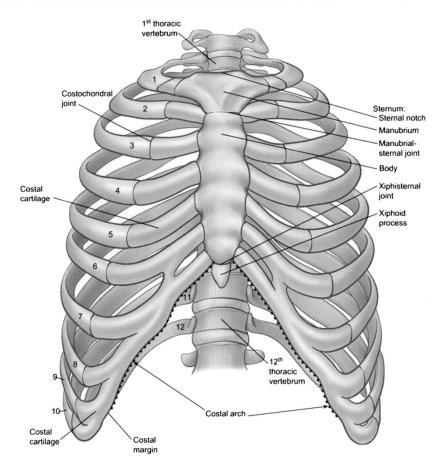

1st thoracic vertebrum

Costochondral joint

Sternum: Sternal notch
Manubrium
Manubrial-sternal joint
Body

Costal cartilage

Xiphisternal joint

Xiphoid process

12th thoracic vertebrum

Costal arch

Costal cartilage   Costal margin

Fig. 8.1 Anatomy of the anterior chest wall. (From Son MBF, Sundel RP. Musculoskeletal causes of pediatric chest pain. *Pediatr Clin N Am*. 2010;57(6):1385–1395 [Fig. 1]. ISSN 0031-3955, https://doi.org/10.1016/j.pcl.2010.09.011, http://www.sciencedirect.com/science/article/pii/S0031395510001586.)

Ribs 8, 9, and 10 attach to the costal cartilage of the rib directly above. The cartilages of ribs 11 and 12 are called floating ribs because they end in the abdominal musculature (see Fig. 8.1). The muscles of the anterior chest wall may also serve as a nidus of atypical chest pain (Fig. 8.2).

CLINICAL SYNDROME

Precordial catch syndrome, also known as Texidor twinge, is a common cause of chest wall pain. Occurring most frequently in adolescents and young adults, precordial catch syndrome is the cause of anxiety among patients and clinicians alike, given the intensity of the pain and its frequent attribution to the heart.

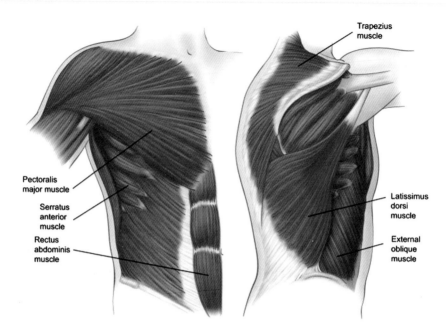

Fig. 8.2 Muscles of the anterior chest wall. (From Son MBF, Sundel RP. Musculoskeletal causes of pediatric chest pain. *Pediatr Clin N Am*. 2010;57(6):1385–1395 [Fig. 2]. ISSN 0031-3955, https://doi.org/10.1016/j.pcl.2010.09.011, http://www.sciencedirect.com/science/article/pii/S0031395510001586.)

Precordial catch syndrome almost always occurs at rest, often while the patient is sitting in a slumped position on an old couch (Fig. 8.3). Distinct from other causes of chest wall pain, precordial catch syndrome is characterized by sharp, stabbing, needlelike pain that is well localized in the precordial region (Table 8.1). It often is perceived at the left sternal border, reinforcing the belief that the pain is cardiac in origin. Symptoms begin without warning, only adding to the patient's anxiety, and they go away as suddenly as they came. The pain lasts from 30 seconds to 3 minutes, and it is often made worse by deep inspiration. Patients suffering from precordial catch syndrome usually outgrow the syndrome by the third decade of life.

SIGNS AND SYMPTOMS

No physical findings (e.g., flushing, pallor, diaphoresis) are associated with the onset of pain, although some patients suffering from precordial catch syndrome may demonstrate tenderness to palpation in the anterior intercostal muscles overlying the painful area. Because the pain is made worse with deep inspiration, the patient may become lightheaded from prolonged shallow breathing.

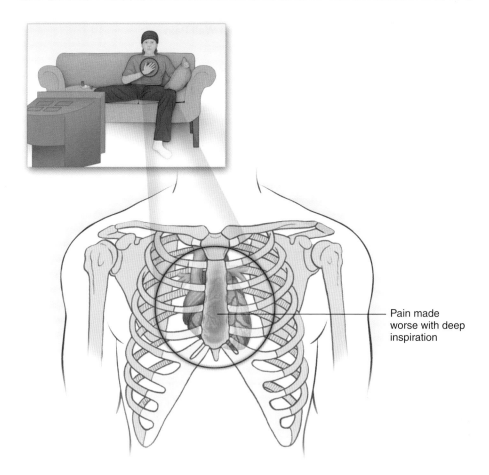

Pain made
worse with deep
inspiration

Fig. 8.3 Precordial catch syndrome can be caused by prolonged sitting in a slumped position. It is often confused with pain of cardiac origin. (From Waldman S. *Atlas of Common Pain Syndromes*. ed. 4. Philadelphia: Elsevier; 2019 [Fig. 66-1].)

TESTING

Plain radiographs are indicated for all patients who present with pain thought to be emanating from the chest wall to rule out occult bony disorders, including tumor. If trauma is present, radionuclide bone scanning should be considered to exclude occult fractures of the ribs or sternum (Fig. 8.4). Given the location of the pain, an ECG and an echocardiogram are indicated, but in patients with precordial catch syndrome, the results are expected to be normal. In patients where the index of suspicion of a cardiac etiology of the patient's symptomatology is high, cardiac stress tests, and in selected cases coronary artery angiography, is indicated. Based on the patient's clinical presentation, additional testing may be

TABLE 8.1 ■ Anatomic Basis of Anterior Chest Wall Pain

Skeleton	Trauma
	Stress fractures (ribs or sternum)
	Chest wall deformities
	Chronic recurrent multifocal osteomyelitis
	SAPHO syndrome
	Precordial catch syndrome
	Hyperalgesia
Joints	Costochondritis
	Tietze syndrome
	Spondyloarthropathies (i.e., psoriatic arthritis)
	Hyperalgesia
Muscles	Muscle strains
	Viral myalgias
	Muscle contusions
	Hyperalgesia
Nerves	Slipping rib syndrome
	Intercostal neuralgia
	Hyperalgesia
Skin	Herpes zoster
	Hyperalgesia

Modified from Son MBF, Sundel RP. Musculoskeletal causes of pediatric chest pain. *Pediatr Clin N Am*. 2010;57(6):1385–1395.

indicated, including a complete blood count, prostate-specific antigen level, erythrocyte sedimentation rate, and antinuclear antibody testing. Magnetic resonance imaging, computed tomography scanning, and ultrasound imaging of the painful area are indicated if an occult mass is suspected and to identify occult pathology (Fig. 8.5).

DIFFERENTIAL DIAGNOSIS

Many other painful conditions that affect the chest wall occur with much greater frequency than precordial catch syndrome (Box 8.1). The costosternal joints are susceptible to osteoarthritis, rheumatoid arthritis, ankylosing spondylitis, Reiter syndrome, and psoriatic arthritis. The joints are often traumatized during acceleration-deceleration injuries and blunt trauma to the chest; with severe trauma, the joints may subluxate or dislocate. Overuse or misuse can result in acute inflammation of the costosternal joint, which can be quite debilitating. The joints are also subject to tumor invasion from primary malignant tumors, including thymoma, or from metastatic disease. Sharp pleuritic chest pain may be associated with devil's grip, pleurisy, pneumonia, or pulmonary embolus. Occult cardiac disease can also mimic the pain of precordial catch syndrome (Fig. 8.6).

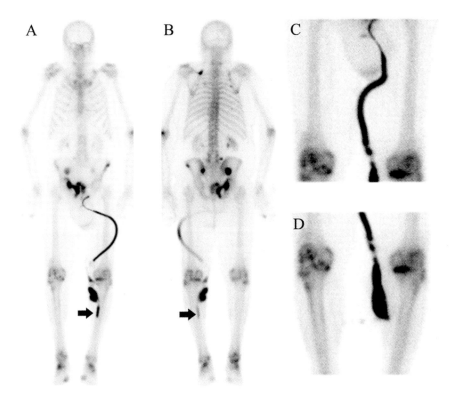

Fig. 8.4 The bone scan study of a patient with prostate cancer showed multiple foci of abnormal tracer uptake in the left scapula, ribs, lower lumbar spine, and pelvic bones consistent with metastases. (A and B) Note is made of urinary catheter with tracer in the urine. The tracer activity projected over the left tibia *(arrow)* is owing to tracer activity in the urinary catheter as shown in the separate static images (C and D) acquired after changing the position of the catheter. This can be misinterpreted as metastasis in the tibia and additional views may be needed. (From Agrawal K, Marafi F, Gnanasegaran G, et al. Pitfalls and limitations of radionuclide planar and hybrid bone imaging. *Sem Nuclear Med.* 2015;45(5):347–372 [Fig. 19]. ISSN 0001-2998, https://doi.org/10.1053/j.semnuclmed. 2015.02.002, http://www.sciencedirect.com/science/article/pii/S0001299815000197.)

TREATMENT

Treatment of precordial catch syndrome consists of a combination of reassurance and instructing the patient to take a deep breath as soon as the pain begins, even though this produces a sharp, stabbing pain. Improving one's posture and changing position frequently while resting or watching television should also help decrease the frequency of attacks. Pharmacologic treatment is not indicated, given the rapid onset and offset of the pain. Significant underlying anxiety caused by concern for the unresolved pain symptomatology should be evaluated and treated appropriately.

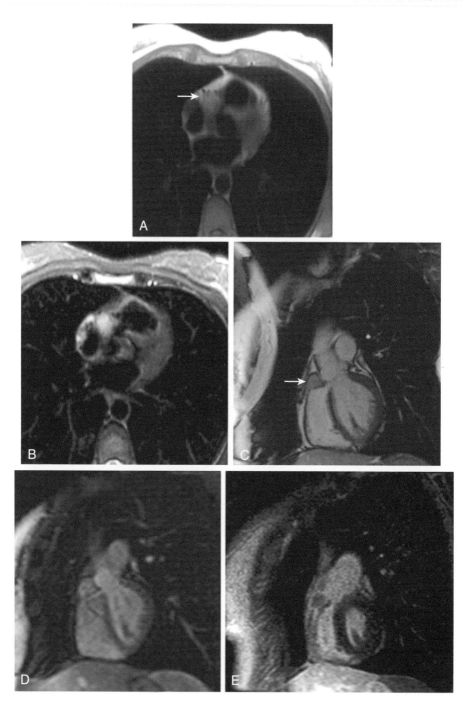

BOX 8.1 ■ Differential Diagnosis of Precordial Catch Syndrome

- Angina
- Cardiac ischemia
- Aortic stenosis
- Mitral valve prolapse
- Pericarditis
- Cardiomyopathy
- Pleuritis
- Devil's grip
- Pleurodynia
- Pulmonary embolus
- Pneumonia
- Rib fractures
- Rib tumors
- Costosternal syndrome
- Manubriosternal joint disorders

PITFALLS AND COMPLICATIONS

Because many pathologic processes may mimic the pain of precordial catch syndrome, the clinician must carefully rule out underlying cardiac disease and diseases of the lung and structures of the mediastinum. Failure to do so could lead to disastrous results. The greatest risk in patients suffering from precordial catch syndrome is related to unnecessary testing (e.g., cardiac catheterization) to rule out cardiac disease.

HIGH-YIELD TAKEAWAYS

- The patient's symptomatology was not associated with antecedent trauma.
- The pain was paroxysmal with pain-free episodes.
- The pain located in the left parasternal region was attributed to a cardiac origin by the patient.
- The patient admitted to increased anxiety and fear regarding the pain.

(Continued)

◄ **Fig. 8.5** Magnetic resonance imaging demonstrating a paraganglioma in the right atrioventricular (AV) groove. (A) Axial T1-weighted image demonstrates an isointense mass *(arrow)* in the right AV groove, immediately subjacent to the right coronary artery. Many of the imaging features of paragangliomas are a result of their high vascularity. (From Syed IS, Feng D, Harris SR, et al. MR imaging of cardiac masses. *Magn Reson Imaging Clin N Am*. 2008;16(2):137–164.) (B) This vascularity gives them a characteristic lightbulb-bright appearance on T2-weighted images. (From Syed IS, Feng D, Harris SR, et al. MR imaging of cardiac masses. *Magn Reson Imaging Clin N Am*. 2008;16(2):137–164.) (C) Coronal steady-state free precession image shows a hyperintense mass in the right AV groove *(arrow)*, again a result of hypervascularity. (D) Paragangliomas appear as hypervascular structures on first-pass perfusion imaging. (E) Delayed enhancement (DE) inversion recovery image demonstrates mild contrast retention but no real DE.

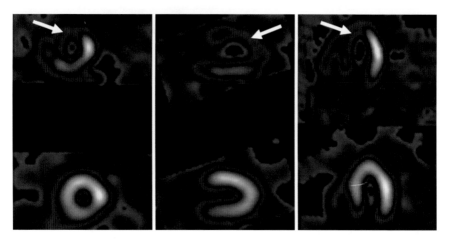

Fig. 8.6 Reversible perfusion defect in the area of an anterior wall and a septum of the left ventricle (probably in the territory of the left anterior descending coronary artery). Upper row: stress perfusion; lower row: rest perfusion. Short-axis slice on the left, vertical long-axis slice in the middle, and horizontal long-axis slice on the right. Images performed with 99mTc methoxyisobutyl isonitrile using single photon emission computed tomography technique. (From Lang O. Radionuclide imaging in acute coronary syndromes. *Cor et Vasa*. 2014;56(4):e354–e361 [Fig. 1]. ISSN 0010-8650, https://doi.org/10.1016/j.crvasa. 2014.04.008, http://www.sciencedirect.com/science/article/pii/S0010865014000472.)

- The patient's pain is not associated with any of the classic symptoms of myocardial ischemia.
- There is no evidence of thrombophlebitis.
- There is no evidence of mitral valve prolapse.
- There are no findings of chest wall or pulmonary pathology that would explain the patient's pain.
- The patient is afebrile, making an acute infectious etiology unlikely.
- All testing is negative, including cardiac stress echocardiography.

Suggested Readings

Ayloo A, Cvengros T, Marella S. Evaluation and treatment of musculoskeletal chest pain. *Prim Care Clin Off Pract*. 2013;40(4):863–887.

Hillen TJ, Wessell DE. Multidetector CT scan in the evaluation of chest pain of nontraumatic musculoskeletal origin. *Thorac Surg Clin*. 2010;20(1):167–173.

Son MBF, Sundel RP. Musculoskeletal causes of pediatric chest pain. *Pediatr Clin North Am*. 2010;57(6):1385–1395.

Stochkendahl MJ, Christensen HW. Chest pain in focal musculoskeletal disorders. *Med Clin North Am*. 2010;94(2):259–273.

Waldman SD. Precordial catch syndrome. In: *Atlas of Common Pain Syndromes*. ed. 4. Philadelphia: Elsevier; 2019:257–259.

Mike Zuckerburg

A 28-Year-Old Male With a Fever and Pleuritic Chest Pain of Acute Onset

- Learn the common causes of chest pain.
- Learn the common causes of hand deformity.
- Develop an understanding of the unique anatomy of the chest wall.
- Develop an understanding of the differential diagnosis of devil's grip.
- Learn to identify the underlying diseases associated with devil's grip.
- Learn the clinical presentation of devil's grip.
- Learn how to examine the chest and chest wall.
- Learn how to use physical examination to identify devil's grip.
- Develop an understanding of the treatment options for devil's grip.

Mike Zuckerburg

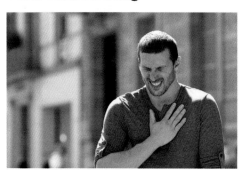

Mike Zuckerburg is a 28-year-old computer technician with the chief complaint of, "I am sicker than a dog." Mike explained, "Everyone in my office is sick; and here it is, the end of summer, but I got it the worst. I can barely get a breath in, it hurts so bad. Doc, I literally cannot take a deep breath. Do you think I have pneumonia? I really feel punk." Mike was a longstanding patient of the practice. One of the retired partners had delivered him and taken care of him until retirement, and I added Mike to my patient list. Mike stated that he had what he thought was a summer cold. It seemed that everybody in the office got sick at once, but over the last couple of days, he became increasingly sicker with a cough and severe pain every time he took a breath.

Mike noted that the pain was worse with coughing, deep breathing, or any movement of the chest wall. He tried using a heating pad and extra-strength Tylenol without much success. I asked about Motrin, but he said it "ate a hole in my stomach. Doc, what do you think is going on here? I think this is about the sickest I have ever been." I could see that Mike looked systemically ill, and it was obvious that he was really worried. I tried to reassure him that we would figure it out.

Mike denied any antecedent chest wall trauma, or pulmonary or cardiac disease. I asked what made the pain better and he said, "Nothing really helps. I spend all my time trying to not cough or breathe too deeply because it hurts so much." Mike said he had a fever for the last couple of days, usually around 100; the highest was 100.6. "I didn't have chills, but I don't have much of an appetite, a little diarrhea. I really don't feel good." I asked Mike to describe his pain, and he said it felt like someone was sticking a knife in his chest and twisting it each time he took a breath. "It feels like I've got a stitch or a catch every time I breathe. I am sleeping in my recliner so I can get a little rest. It just hurts too much to lie down."

On physical examination, Mike had a mild fever at 100.2 orally. His respirations were 18, and his pulse was 86 and regular. He was normotensive with a blood pressure of 126/74. Mike's oxygen saturation on room air was 98%. His head, eyes, ears, nose, throat (HEENT) exam was unremarkable, nothing to suggest strep throat. His cardiac exam was completely normal. Peripheral pulses were full. His pulmonary exam was a different story. He had a loud friction rub anteriorly on the left. It was easy to hear, even over all of the upper airway secretions he had from not coughing. His thyroid was normal, and there was no adenopathy. His abdominal examination revealed no abnormal mass or organomegaly. There was no costovertebral angle (CVA) tenderness or peripheral edema. Mike's low back examination was unremarkable. Visual inspection of the chest wall was unremarkable with no costochondral swelling or costochondritis. Examination of his major joints revealed no acute arthritis. A careful neurologic examination revealed no evidence of peripheral or entrapment neuropathy, and the deep tendon reflexes were normal. There was no evidence of thrombophlebitis.

Key Clinical Points—What's Important and What's Not

THE HISTORY

- History of acute onset of fever and right-sided pleuritic chest pain
- History of multiple coworkers suffering from a febrile illness
- No history of previous significant chest pain
- Mild fever for 48 hours
- No history of chills
- Exacerbation of pain with coughing, movement of the chest wall, and deep breathing
- Sleep disturbance

THE PHYSICAL EXAMINATION

- Patient is febrile
- Normal oxygen saturation on room air
- Minimal findings on physical examination of the chest wall
- Cardiac examination is normal
- Presence of a loud friction rub over the left anterior chest wall
- No evidence of infection
- Pain elicited on deep inspiration

OTHER FINDINGS OF NOTE

- Normal HEENT examination
- Normal abdominal examination
- No peripheral edema
- Normal upper extremity neurologic examination, motor and sensory examination
- Examinations of major joints were normal
- No evidence of thrombophlebitis

🔬 What Tests Would You Like to Order?

The following tests were ordered:

- Chest x-ray
- Electrocardiogram (ECG)

TEST RESULTS

The plain radiograph of the chest revealed a small pleural effusion on the left (Fig. 9.1).

The ECG is reported as normal (Fig. 9.2).

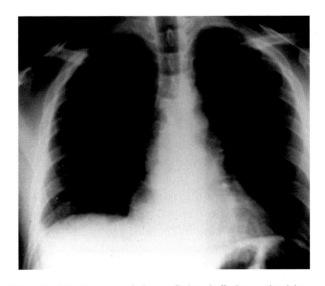

Fig. 9.1   Plain radiograph of the chest revealed a small pleural effusion on the right.

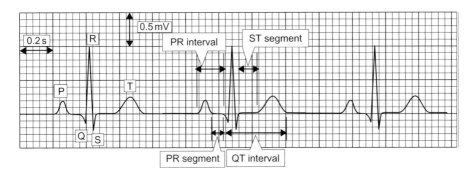

Fig. 9.2   Normal electrocardiogram. (From Feher J. *Quantitative Human Physiology*. Waltham: Academic Press; 2012 [Fig. 5.6.3].)

Clinical Correlation—Putting It All Together

What is the diagnosis?
- Devil's grip (Bornholm disease)

The Science Behind the Diagnosis

ANATOMY

The outer parietal pleura and inner pleura work together to help decrease the effort of breathing by allowing the two layers of pleura to slide against each other (Fig. 9.3). Between the two pleurae lies the pleural cavity, which contains a small amount of pleural fluid that facilitates this sliding function. The pleural fluid also helps maintain surface tension adequate to allow the visceral pleura to adhere closely to the parietal pleura, thus optimizing expansion of the lungs. The outer visceral pleura is tightly attached to the chest wall, while the inner visceral pleura covers the lungs and adjacent structures. The parietal pleura is highly sensitive to pain with its costal and cervical surfaces as well as the outer diaphragmatic surfaces innervated by the intercostal nerves. The more central diaphragmatic and mediastinal surfaces of the parietal pleura are innervated by the phrenic nerve (Fig. 9.4). The visceral pleura receives no somatic sensory innervation, but it is innervated by the autonomic nervous system. The blood supply of the parietal pleura is from the intercostal arteries, with the visceral pleura receiving its blood supply directly from bronchial circulation. Contraction of the external intercostal muscles and the hemidiaphragms causes expansion of the chest wall resulting in an increased lung volume. This increased lung volume creates a negative pressure within the airways causing inspiration to occur. Relaxation of these muscles decreases the lung volume causing expiration. During periods of heavy respiration, the sternocleidomastoid and scalene muscles may serve as accessory respiratory muscles.

CLINICAL SYNDROME

Devil's grip is an uncommon cause of chest pain. Also known as Bornholm disease, the grip of the phantom, dry pleurisy, acute epidemic pleurodynia, and Sylvest disease, devil's grip is caused by acute infection with coxsackievirus (Box 9.1). This virus is transmitted via the fecal-oral route and is highly contagious, owing to a long period of viral shedding of 6 weeks. In some patients, their immune system limits the infection to a mild fever or flulike illness called summer fever. In others, a full-fledged infection with resultant pleurodynia and cough develops.

Devil's grip has a seasonal variation in occurrence, with 90% of cases occurring in the summer and fall, with August being the peak month. No gender predilection is seen, but the disease occurs more commonly in young adults and

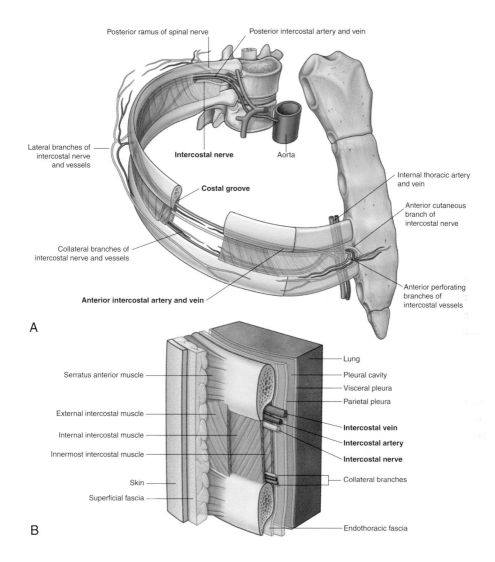

Fig. 9.3 The pleura and contents of the intercostal space. (A) Oblique coronal view of the anatomy of the intercostal nerve and vessels. (B) Cross-section through two adjacent ribs demonstrating the relationship of the intercostal muscles, ribs, pleura, and intercostal nerve, artery, and vein. (C) Coronal view demonstrating the relationship of the lungs, mediastinum, sternum, and ribs. (From Drake R, Vogl W, Mitchell A. *Gray's Anatomy for Students*. ed. 4. Philadelphia: Churchill Livingstone; 2020 [Fig. 3.26].)

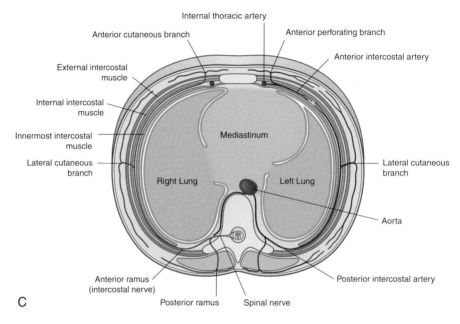

C

Fig. 9.3 Continued.

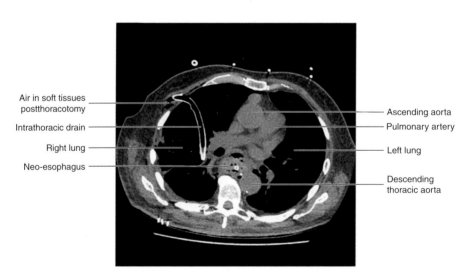

Fig 9.4 Axial CT demonstrating the relationship of the ribs, contents of the mediastium, and lungs in a post-thoracotmy patient. Note air in the soft tissues. (From Drake R, Vogl W, Mitchell A. *Gray's Anatomy for Students*. ed. 4. Philadelphia: Churchill Livingstone; 2020 [Fig. 3.33].)

BOX 9.1 ■ Various Names for Devil's Grip

- Devil's grip
- Devil's grippe
- Summer fever
- Bornholm disease
- Phantom's grip
- Dry pleurisy
- Acute epidemic pleurodynia
- Sylvest disease

---

occasionally in children. The pain is severe and described as sharp or pleuritic. The pain occurs in paroxysms that can last 30 minutes.

SIGNS AND SYMPTOMS

Physical examination of a patient with devil's grip reveals the appearance of acute illness (Fig. 9.5). Pallor and fever are invariably present, as is tachycardia. Patients may report malaise, sore throat, and arthralgia, which may confuse the clinical picture. Examination of the chest wall reveals minimal physical findings, although a friction rub is sometimes present. During the paroxysms of pain, the patient suffering from devil's grip attempts to splint or protect the affected area. Deep inspiration or movement of the chest wall markedly increases the pain of devil's grip.

TESTING

Plain radiographs are indicated in all patients with pain thought to be the result of infection with coxsackievirus to rule out occult chest wall pathology, pulmonary tumors, pneumonia, or empyema (Figs. 9.6 and 9.7). Ventilation-perfusion studies of the lungs are indicated if pulmonary embolism is being considered in the differential diagnosis. Based on the patient's clinical presentation, additional tests (complete blood cell count, sedimentation rate, and throat cultures for Streptococcus) may be indicated. Computed tomography (CT) scan of the thoracic contents is indicated if occult mass or empyema is suspected (Fig. 9.8). Ultrasound imaging can be useful in diagnosing occult pneumothorax (Fig. 9.9).

DIFFERENTIAL DIAGNOSIS

As is the case with costochondritis, costosternal joint pain, Tietze syndrome, and rib fractures, many patients with devil's grip first seek medical attention because

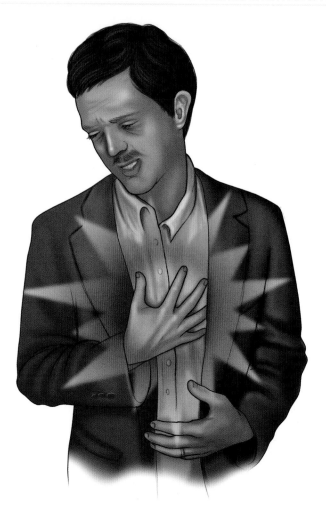

Fig. 9.5 The patient suffering from devil's grip appears acutely ill, and this disease diagnosis should be considered in the differential diagnosis of any patient with an acute febrile illness and pleuritic chest pain. (From Waldman S. *Atlas of Uncommon Pain Syndromes*. ed. 4. Philadelphia: Elsevier; 2020 [Fig. 65-1].)

they believe they are having a heart attack. If the area innervated by the subcostal nerve is involved, patients may believe they have gallbladder disease. Statistically, children with devil's grip have abdominal pain more often than do adults, and such pain may be attributed to appendicitis, leading to unnecessary surgery. In contradistinction to most other causes of pain involving the chest wall, which are musculoskeletal or neuropathic, the pain of devil's grip is infectious. The constitutional symptoms associated with devil's grip may lead the clinician to consider pneumonia, empyema, and occasionally pulmonary embolus as the most likely diagnosis.

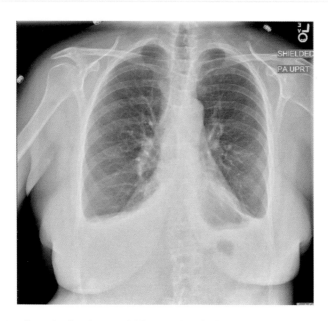

Fig. 9.6 Chest radiograph showing small bilateral pleural effusions with no airspace disease in a patient with devil's grip. (From Lal A, Akhtar J, Isaac S, et al. Unusual cause of chest pain, Bornholm disease, a forgotten entity; case report and review of literature. *Resp Med Case Rep.* 2018;25:270—273 [Fig. 2]. ISSN 2213-0071, https://doi.org/10.1016/j.rmcr.2018.10.005, http://www.sciencedirect.com/science/article/pii/S2213007118302338.)

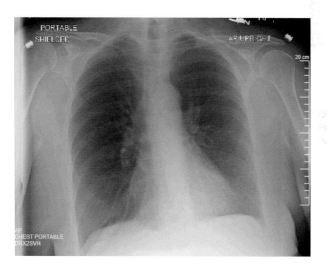

Fig. 9.7 Chest radiograph repeated of the same patient as in Fig. 9.6 after 2 weeks showing complete resolution of pleural effusions. (From Lal A, Akhtar J, Isaac S, et al. Unusual cause of chest pain, Bornholm disease, a forgotten entity; case report and review of literature. *Resp Med Case Rep.* 2018;25:270—273 [Fig. 3]. ISSN 2213-0071, https://doi.org/10.1016/j.rmcr.2018.10.005, http://www.sciencedirect.com/science/article/pii/S2213007118302338.)

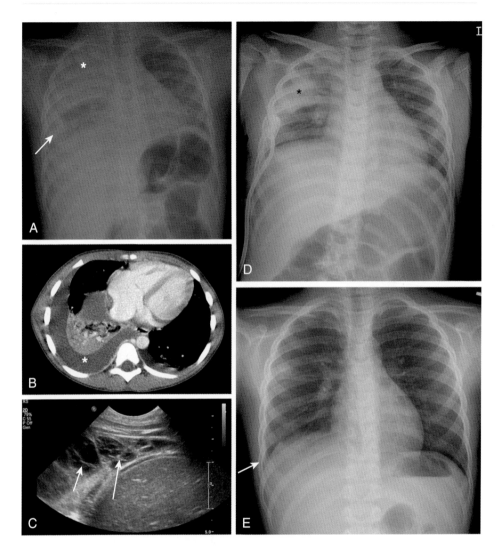

Fig. 9.8 This patient presented with a right upper lobe pneumonia *(*)* and a pleural effusion *(arrow)* (A). (B) Chest computed tomography shows the effusion *(*)* that appears to be free-flowing, as it is dependent. (C) An ultrasound shows multiple septations in the pleural fluid *(arrows)*. (D) Radiograph after image-guided insertion of a small-bore chest tube and fibrinolytic therapy. The empyema is nearly resolved, with persistent pneumonia *(*)* causing persistent fevers. (E) Minimal residual pleural thickening *(arrow)* seen after removal of the chest tube and completion of antibiotics. (From Hogan MJ, Coley BD. Interventional radiology treatment of empyema and lung abscesses. *Paediatr Respir Rev.* 2008;9:77–84.)

As mentioned earlier, the pain of devil's grip is often mistaken for pain of cardiac or gallbladder origin and can lead to visits to the emergency department and unnecessary cardiac and gastrointestinal workups. If trauma has occurred, devil's grip may coexist with fractured ribs or fractures of the sternum itself,

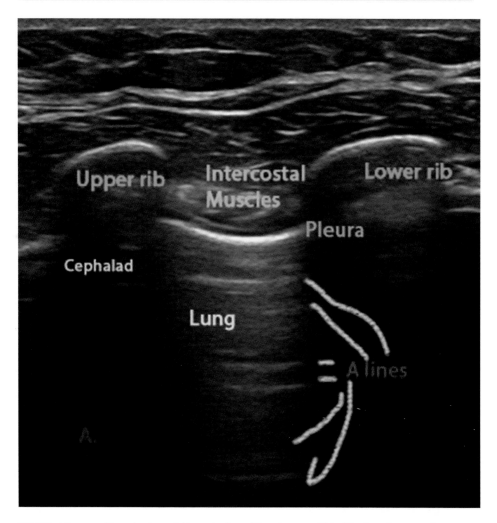

Fig. 9.9 Ultrasound imaging is useful in evaluation of the pleura and identification of pneumothorax.

which can be missed on plain radiographs and may require radionuclide bone scanning for proper identification. Tietze syndrome, which is painful enlargement of the upper costochondral cartilage associated with viral infection, can be confused with devil's grip.

Neuropathic pain involving the chest wall also may be confused or coexist with costosternal syndrome. Examples of such neuropathic pain include diabetic polyneuropathies and acute herpes zoster involving the thoracic nerves. The possibility of diseases of the structures of the mediastinum is ever present, and such disease sometimes can be difficult to diagnose. Pathologic processes that inflame the pleura, such as pulmonary embolus, infection, and tumor, also need to be considered.

TREATMENT

Initial treatment of devil's grip should include a combination of simple analgesics and nonsteroidal antiinflammatory drugs or cyclooxygenase-2 inhibitors. If these medications do not control the patient's symptoms adequately, opioid analgesics may be added during the period of acute pain. Local application of heat and cold also may be beneficial to provide symptomatic relief of the pain of devil's grip. The use of an elastic rib belt may help provide symptomatic relief in some patients.

For patients who do not respond to the aforementioned treatment modalities, consideration should be given to intercostal nerve block using a local anesthetic and steroid in the most painful area.

HIGH-YIELD TAKEAWAYS

- The patient is febrile, making an acute infectious etiology (e.g., pneumonia) a prime consideration.
- The seasonal variation of devil's grip is consistent with peak illness occurring in late summer and early fall.
- The patient's symptomatology is consistent with devil's grip.
- Given the seriousness of the many diseases that can cause pleuritic chest pain, devil's grip must be considered a diagnosis of exclusion.
- Plain radiographs will provide high-yield information regarding the bony contents of the chest wall, but CT scanning, ultrasound imaging, and magnetic resonance imaging will be more useful in helping rule out diseases that may mimic the clinical presentation of devil's grip.

Suggested Readings

Connolly JH, O'Neill HJ. Bornholm disease associated with coxsackie A9 virus infection. *Lancet*. 1971;298(7732):1035.

Cotterill JA. The devil's grip. *Lancet*. 1973;301(7815):1308–1309.

Ikeda RM, Kondracki SF, Drabkin PD, et al. Pleurodynia among football players at a high school: an outbreak associated with coxsackievirus B1. *JAMA*. 1993;270:2205–2206.

Stalkup JR, Chilukuri S. Enterovirus infections: a review of clinical presentation, diagnosis, and treatment. *Dermatol Clin*. 2002;20(2):217–223.

Waldman SD. Devil's grip. In: *Atlas of Uncommon Pain Syndromes*. ed. 4. Philadelphia: Elsevier; 2019:219–222.

Tommy "Tank" Teller

A 68-Year-Old Diabetic With Pain and Paresthesias Radiating Into the Lower Chest and Subcostal Area

- Learn the common causes of chest wall and subcostal pain.
- Learn the common causes of chest wall and subcostal numbness.
- Develop an understanding of the impact of diabetes on the peripheral nerves.
- Develop an understanding of the anatomy of the intercostal and subcostal nerves.
- Develop an understanding of the causes of peripheral neuropathy.
- Develop an understanding of the differential diagnosis of chest wall and subcostal pain.
- Learn the clinical presentation of diabetic truncal neuropathy.
- Learn how to examine the thoracic dermatomes.
- Learn how to use physical examination to identify diabetic truncal neuropathy.
- Develop an understanding of the treatment options for diabetic truncal neuropathy.

Tommy Teller

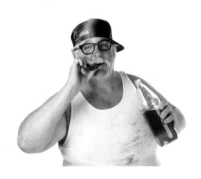

Tommy "Tank" Teller is a 68-year-old motorcycle mechanic. He begins our visit by saying, "What the hell, Doc? Don't let anybody tell you that getting old is any fun. It's been one thing after another, first the cataracts and now this." I asked him, "What's the problem, Tank?" Tommy retorts, "Doc, are you blind? Here you are asking me what's the problem. Are you kidding? And to think, I'm here in my best T-shirt and all." It was all I could do to keep from laughing. Tommy was never one for sartorial splendor, but today he was looking particularly "tanklike." Tommy has been a patient of mine for the last few years. He is a really good guy but not a picture of health. I first saw Tommy when his ophthalmologist asked me to clear him for cataract surgery. The whole thing started when he had failed his eye test when trying to renew his driver's license. I remember that as I was introducing myself to Tommy, he shook my hand and said, "Doc, fat, stupid, and blind is no way to go through life. But at least we can fix one of them." Other than cataract surgery a couple of years ago, Tommy said he hadn't seen a doctor since he had to get his hand stitched up about 10 years ago. As I quickly figured out, fat, stupid, and blind were just the beginning of Tommy's list. We had to add hypertension and poorly controlled type 2 diabetes. I had done my best to get Tommy tuned up for his surgery, and we got him through it without too much drama. As I got to know Tommy, I realized that the "good old boy" persona was just an act. He was actually a pretty interesting guy. He knew something about most anything I mentioned. Tommy's problem lies with compliance—and the lack thereof. In spite of my best efforts, his blood pressure and blood sugar were poorly controlled at the best of times. I could hardly wait to see what his current situation involved. As I was thinking about this, Tommy pulled his T-shirt over his head, and I immediately saw the answer.

"Don't you think I'm getting a little old to be pregnant? I took all the precautions and now this," said Tommy as he pointed to the large bulge poking out of the right side of his abdomen (Fig. 10.1). "When did that show up?" I asked. Tommy said, "Hank—you know, after Hank Williams—has been there for about a month. Doc, I've had a good life. Do you think I have the big C? One of the guys I work with says too much drinking can mess with your liver, but he didn't say it would get you pregnant! What the hell, Doc? I would be lying if I said I wasn't scared."

I asked Tommy how his blood sugars had been doing, and he give me a sheepish grin and said that he had been meaning to get by the drugstore to get

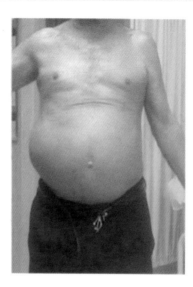

Fig. 10.1 With significant motor involvement of the subcostal nerve, a patient suffering from diabetic truncal neuropathy may complain that the abdomen bulges outward. (From Waldman S. *Atlas of Common Pain Syndromes*. ed. 4. Philadelphia: Elsevier; 2019 [Fig. 64-2].)

some test strips, but he had been awfully busy of late. I responded, "So I take that to mean that you haven't been checking your sugars. What about your high blood pressure pills?" Tommy said that he took them when he remembered, but added, "They mess with my willy so if I *have plans*, I don't take them." I shook my head and thought, "This guy is going to kill himself if he keeps on." I asked Tommy to describe any numbness associated with his "pregnancy," and he said that he had "weird needles and pins sensation over the baby bump" that drove him crazy and kept him up at night.

I asked Tommy about any fever, chills, or other constitutional symptoms such as weight loss, jaundice, night sweats, etc., and he shook his head no. He denied any recent trauma to the abdominal wall or anything else that might account for his symptoms.

I asked Tommy to point with one finger to show me where the pins and needles were, and he pointed to the right subcostal area and said, "Right here, over Hank." Tommy went on to say that he knew it was a boy and gave out a short laugh, but I could tell that he was really scared and was kidding around to cover it up.

On physical examination, Tommy was afebrile. His respirations were 16, his pulse was 72 and regular, and his blood pressure was 168/90. In his T-shirt and underwear, Tommy weighed 268 pounds, up 10 pounds from his last visit. His fundoscopic examination was a mess. He had most everything wrong you could see on a patient's retina (Fig. 10.2). "So, Tank, when is the last time you saw the eye

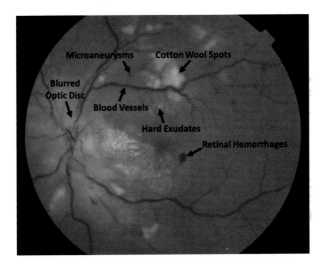

Fig. 10.2 Image of a retina demonstrating the sequelae of poorly controlled diabetes and hypertension. (From Akram MU, Akbar A, Hassan T, et al. Data on fundus images for vessels segmentation, detection of hypertensive retinopathy, diabetic retinopathy and papilledema. *Data Brief.* 2020;29:105282 [Fig. 1]. ISSN 2352-3409, https://doi.org/10.1016/j.dib.2020.105282, http://www.sciencedirect.com/science/article/pii/S2352340920301761.)

doctor?" "You remember, Doc! It's when I got my cataracts fixed—must be about 2 years ago." I shook my head and continued to examine the patient. The rest of his head, eyes, ears, nose, throat (HEENT) exam was normal. Because Tommy was one of those guys who liked to chew on a cigar while he was working, I took extra care when I examined his oral mucosa, but things looked pretty good. Other than the hypertension, his cardiac examination was normal. His lungs were clear, and his thyroid was normal. His abdominal examination revealed a large bulge in the subcostal area. It was soft, and there was no abnormal mass or organomegaly. I asked Tommy to suck in his gut, and there was obvious weakness of the abdominal wall muscles on the right. His eyes weren't the only thing that the diabetes got, I thought, as I completed my exam. There was no costovertebral angle (CVA) tenderness. There was no peripheral edema, and his peripheral pulses were 1+. A careful examination of his feet revealed no diabetic ulcers, and his nail care was good. His low back examination was unremarkable. Visual inspection of the skin over his right subcostal region revealed no evidence of current or past herpes zoster infection, and the skin was otherwise unremarkable. There was no rubor or color. There was no obvious abdominal wall hernia. A careful neurologic examination of the upper extremities revealed a symmetric decrease in sensation distally in all four extremities, consistent with diabetic neuropathy. "Tank, I think that the diabetes has got your nerves. You may want to change Hank's name to Sugar, because if you don't get your blood sugars and your blood pressure under control, Hank is going to be the least of your problems." He replied, "I hear you, Doc . . . I hear you,

Doc." I shook my head and wondered if Tank ever heard anything I said. Oh well, my job was to keep trying, and I knew that I would.

Key Clinical Points—What's Important and What's Not

THE HISTORY

- History of onset of painless bulging of the abdominal wall in the absence of antecedent trauma
- History of poorly controlled diabetes
- History of obesity
- History of poorly controlled hypertension
- History of onset of right chest wall and subcostal pain with associated paresthesias
- No fever or chills

THE PHYSICAL EXAMINATION

- Patient is afebrile
- Obvious weakness of the right abdominal wall
- Decreased sensation in the distribution of the subcostal nerve
- Grossly abnormal fundoscopic examination
- Findings consistent with symmetric diabetic polyneuropathy
- No evidence of infection
- No evidence of herpes zoster
- Hypertension
- Obesity

OTHER FINDINGS OF NOTE

- Otherwise normal HEENT examination
- Normal cardiac examination
- Normal pulmonary examination
- No abdominal wall hernia
- No organomegaly
- No peripheral edema

What Tests Would You Like to Order?

The following tests were ordered:
- Electromyography (EMG) and nerve conduction velocity testing of the lower thoracic dermatomes and extremities

- Complete chemistry profile
- Hemoglobin A1c (HbA1c) determination
- Urinalysis

TEST RESULTS

EMG and nerve conduction velocity testing revealed a subacute-chronic neurogenic pattern, characterized by complex and long-duration motor unit potentials and increased percentage of polyphasic potentials. Evidence of spontaneous activity, including positive sharp waves, was noted, as well as an associated mixed sensory-motor polyneuropathy in all four extremities.

Tests showed an abnormal complete chemistry profile, including a blood sugar of 282 and an elevated creatinine at 1.5.

There was an elevated HbA1c determination of 10.8.

Abnormal urinalysis showed 1 + proteinuria.

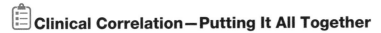

Clinical Correlation—Putting It All Together

What is the diagnosis?
- Diabetic truncal neuropathy

The Science Behind the Diagnosis

ANATOMY

The precise mechanisms responsible for diabetic neuropathy continue to be elucidated, with the current concepts as to the evolution of diabetic neuropathy adopting a multifactorial pathologic approach (Fig. 10.3). Maladaption and dysfunction of the nervous and vascular systems provide the basis for the angiopathy and neural damage that lead to diabetic polyneuropathy. Concurrent inflammatory and immune responses combined with mitrochondrial dysfunction and schwannopathy appear to also play a role in the pathogenesis of diabetic polyneuropathy.

CLINICAL SYNDROME

Diabetic neuropathy is a term used by clinicians to describe a heterogeneous group of diseases that affect the autonomic and peripheral nervous systems of patients suffering from diabetes mellitus (Fig. 10.4). Diabetic neuropathy is now thought to be the most common form of peripheral neuropathy that afflicts humankind, with an estimated 220 million people worldwide suffering from this

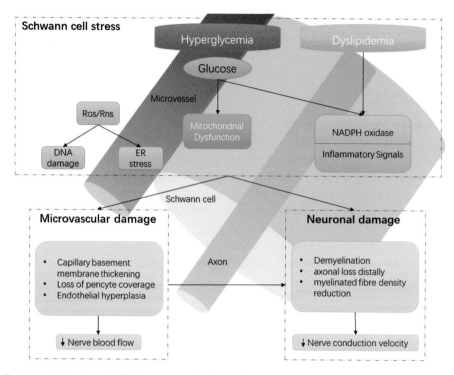

Fig. 10.3 Mechanism of diabetic neuropathy. Hyperglycemia-driven Schwann cell stress and neuronal damage. Hyperglycemia and dyslipidemia ultimately lead to reduction of neuronal support from Schwann cells and microvessels. Disruption of neuronal support by Schwann cells and the vascular system contributes to neuropathy, in conjunction with the direct effects of diabetes on neurons. *ER*, Endoplasmic reticulum; *Ros*, reactive oxygen species; *Rns*, reactive nitrogen species. (From Sloan G, Shillo P, Selvarajah D, et al. A new look at painful diabetic neuropathy. *Diabetes Res Clin Pract*. 2018;144:177–191 [Fig. 1]. ISSN 0168-8227, https://doi.org/10.1016/j.diabres.2018.08.020, http://www.sciencedirect.com/science/article/pii/S0168822718311926.)

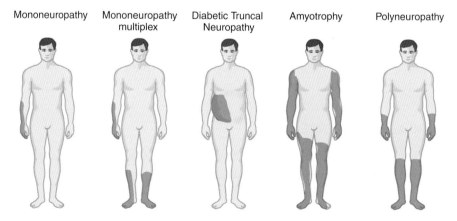

Fig. 10.4 Classifications of diabetic neuropathy.

BOX 10.1 ■ The Impact of Diabetes Mellitus on the Nervous System

Sensorimotor neuropathy
 Distal symmetric polyneuropathy
 Diabetic mononeuropathy
 Carpal tunnel syndrome
 Tarsal tunnel syndrome
 Ulnar neuropathy
 Lateral femoral cutaneous nerve entrapment syndrome
 Focal neuropathy (usually confined to the distribution of a single cranial or peripheral
  nerve)
 Mononeuritis multiplex (can involve the distribution of several peripheral nerves)
 Diabetic amyotrophy
Diabetic autonomic neuropathy
 Hypoglycemic unawareness
 Silent myocardial ischemia
 Orthostatic hypotension and abnormal circadian blood pressures
 Altered exercise tolerance
 Genitourinary
 Neurogenic bladder
 Frequent urinary tract infections
 Urinary incontinence
 Sexual dysfunction
 Gastropathy
 Gastroparesis
 Abdominal pain and bloating
 Diarrhea and constipation
 Fecal incontinence
 Malabsorption
 Dysphagia
 Sudomotor abnormalities
 Gustatory sweating
 Sweating only from the chest down
 High risk of Charcot arthropathy

Modified from Unger J, Cole BE. Recognition and management of diabetic neuropathy. *Prim Care Clin Off Pract.* 2007;34(4):887–913. ISSN 0095-4543, https://doi.org/10.1016/j.pop.2007.07.003, http://www.sciencedirect.com/science/article/pii/S0095454307000632.)

malady. It is important for the clinician to remember that no organ system is spared from the impact that diabetes mellitus has on the nervous system, and there are factors that can be managed to mitigate the impact of the disease (Boxes 10.1 and 10.2).

One of the most commonly encountered forms of diabetic neuropathy is diabetic truncal neuropathy. In this condition, pain and motor dysfunction are often incorrectly attributed to intrathoracic or intraabdominal disorders and lead to extensive workups for appendicitis, cholecystitis, renal calculi, and more. The onset of symptoms frequently coincides with periods of extreme hypoglycemia or hyperglycemia, or with weight loss or gain. Patients who

---

BOX 10.2 ■ Factors That Can Be Modified to Mitigate the Impact of Diabetes Mellitus on the Nervous System

- Decreasing glycemic variability with tight control of blood sugars
- Managing dyslipidemias, including hypertriglyceridemia
- Managing comorbidities, including hypertension
- Managing obesity
- Smoking cessation
- Improving diet
- Treating vitamin deficiencies

---

present with diabetic truncal neuropathy complain of severe dysesthetic pain with patchy sensory deficits in the distribution of the lower thoracic or upper thoracic dermatomes. The pain is often worse at night and causes significant sleep disturbance. The symptoms of diabetic truncal neuropathy often resolve spontaneously over 6 to 12 months; however, because of the severity of symptoms, aggressive treatment with pharmacotherapy and neural blockade is indicated.

SIGNS AND SYMPTOMS

Physical examination generally reveals minimal findings unless the patient has a history of previous thoracic or subcostal surgery or cutaneous evidence of herpes zoster involving the thoracic dermatomes. Unlike patients with musculoskeletal causes of chest wall and subcostal pain, patients with diabetic truncal neuropathy do not attempt to splint or protect the affected area. Careful sensory examination of the affected dermatomes may reveal decreased sensation or allodynia (Fig. 10.5). With significant motor involvement of the subcostal nerve, the patient may complain that the abdomen bulges outward (see Fig. 10.1). This abnormal bulging is known as pseudohernia.

TESTING

The presence of diabetes should lead to a high index of suspicion for diabetic truncal neuropathy. If the diagnosis of diabetic truncal neuropathy is suspected based on the targeted history and physical examination, screening laboratory tests (complete blood count, chemistry profile, HbA1c determination, erythrocyte sedimentation rate, thyroid function studies, antinuclear antibody testing, and urinalysis) should rule out most other peripheral neuropathies that are easily treatable. EMG and nerve conduction velocity testing are indicated in all patients suffering from peripheral neuropathy to identify treatable entrapment neuropathies and further delineate the type of peripheral neuropathy present.

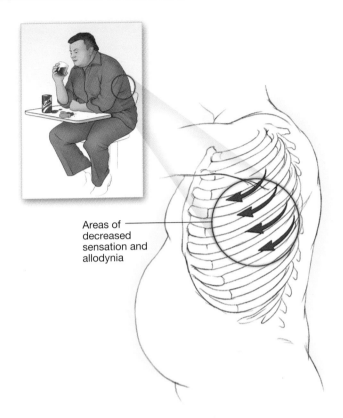

Areas of decreased sensation and allodynia

Fig. 10.5 The pain of diabetic truncal neuropathy is neuropathic and is often made worse by poorly controlled blood glucose levels. (From Waldman S. *Atlas of Common Pain Syndromes*. ed. 4. Philadelphia: Elsevier; 2019 [Fig. 64-1].)

These tests may also be able to quantify the severity of peripheral or entrapment neuropathy. Additional laboratory testing is indicated as the clinical situation dictates (e.g., Lyme disease titers, heavy metal screens). Magnetic resonance imaging of the spinal canal and cord should be performed if myelopathy is suspected. Nerve or skin biopsy is occasionally indicated if no cause of the peripheral neuropathy can be ascertained (Fig. 10.6). Lack of response to the therapies discussed later should lead to a reconsideration of the diagnosis and repetition of testing as clinically indicated.

DIFFERENTIAL DIAGNOSIS

Diseases other than diabetic neuropathy may cause peripheral neuropathies in diabetic patients. These diseases may exist alone or may coexist with diabetic truncal neuropathy, thus making identification and treatment difficult.

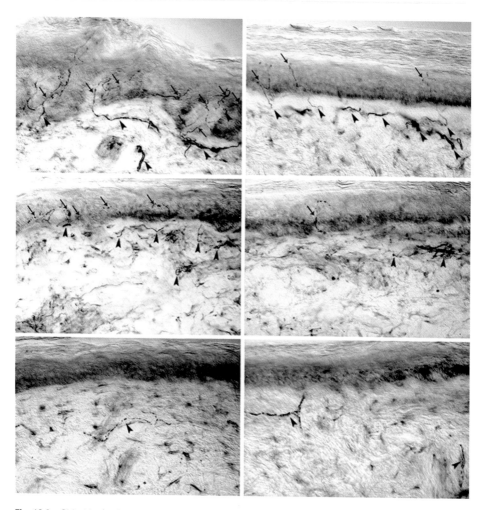

Fig. 10.6 Skin biopsy from the proximal thigh *(left column)* and distal leg *(right column)* with protein gene product 9.5 immunohistochemistry. The pattern of cutaneous innervation is demonstrated in healthy volunteers *(top row)*, a patient with distal symmetric polyneuropathy *(middle row)*, and a patient with sensory neuropathy *(bottom row)*. Arrows indicate intraepidermal nerve fibers, and arrowheads indicate subpapillary nerve bundles. (From Sloan G, Shillo P, Selvarajah D, et al. A new look at painful diabetic neuropathy. *Diabetes Res Clin Pract*. 2018;144:177−191 [Fig. 3]. ISSN 0168-8227, https://doi.org/10.1016/j.diabres.2018.08.020, http://www.sciencedirect.com/science/article/pii/S0168822718311926.)

Although uncommon in the United States, Hansen disease is a common cause of peripheral neuropathy worldwide that may mimic or coexist with diabetic truncal neuropathy. Other infectious causes of peripheral neuropathies include Lyme disease and human immunodeficiency virus infection. Substances that are toxic to nerves, including alcohol, heavy metals, chemotherapeutic agents, and hydrocarbons, may also cause peripheral neuropathies that are indistinguishable from diabetic neuropathy on clinical grounds. Heritable disorders such as Charcot-Marie-Tooth disease and other familial diseases of the peripheral nervous system must also be considered, although treatment options are somewhat limited. Metabolic and endocrine causes of peripheral neuropathy that must be ruled out include vitamin deficiencies, pernicious anemia, hypothyroidism, uremia, and acute intermittent porphyria. Other causes of peripheral neuropathy that may confuse the clinical picture include Guillain-Barré syndrome, amyloidosis, entrapment neuropathies, carcinoid syndrome, paraneoplastic syndromes, and sarcoidosis. Because many of these diseases are treatable, it is imperative that the clinician exclude them before attributing a patient's symptoms solely to diabetes.

Intercostal neuralgia and musculoskeletal causes of chest wall and subcostal pain may also be confused with diabetic truncal neuropathy. In all these conditions, the patient's pain may be erroneously attributed to cardiac or upper abdominal disease, thus leading to unnecessary testing and treatment.

TREATMENT

Control of blood glucose levels

The current thinking is that the better the patient's glycemic control, the less severe the symptoms of diabetic truncal neuropathy. Significant swings in blood glucose levels seem to predispose diabetic patients to the development of clinically significant diabetic truncal neuropathy. Some investigators believe that, although oral hypoglycemic agents control blood glucose levels, they do not protect patients from diabetic truncal neuropathy as well as insulin does. In fact, some patients taking hypoglycemic agents experience a reduction in the symptoms of diabetic truncal neuropathy when they are switched to insulin. The role of the newer pharmacologic agents in the prevention of the complications of diabetes appears promising.

Pharmacologic treatment

Antidepressants

Traditionally, tricyclic antidepressants have been a mainstay in the palliation of pain caused by diabetic truncal neuropathy. Controlled studies have demonstrated the efficacy of amitriptyline, and nortriptyline and desipramine have also proved to be clinically useful. Unfortunately, this class of drugs is associated with significant anticholinergic side effects, including dry mouth, constipation, sedation, and urinary retention. These drugs should be used with caution in patients suffering from glaucoma, cardiac arrhythmia, and prostatism. To minimize side effects and encourage compliance, the physician should start amitriptyline or nortriptyline at a 10-mg dose at bedtime; the dose can then be titrated upward to 25 mg at bedtime as side effects allow. Subsequently, upward titration in 25-mg increments can be carried out each week as side effects allow. Even at lower doses, patients generally report a rapid reduction in sleep disturbance and begin to experience some pain relief in 10 to 14 days. If the patient does not show any reduction in pain as the dose is being titrated upward, the addition of gabapentin alone or in combination with nerve blocks is recommended (see later). The selective serotonin reuptake inhibitors, such as fluoxetine, have also been used to treat the pain of diabetic truncal neuropathy, and although these drugs are better tolerated than are the tricyclic antidepressants they appear to be less efficacious.

Anticonvulsants

Anticonvulsants have long been used to treat neuropathic pain, including that of diabetic truncal neuropathy. Both phenytoin and carbamazepine have been used with varying degrees of success, either alone or in combination with antidepressants. Unfortunately, the side effects of these drugs have limited their clinical usefulness.

The anticonvulsant gabapentin is highly efficacious in the treatment of various painful neuropathic conditions, including postherpetic neuralgia and diabetic truncal neuropathy. Used properly, gabapentin is extremely well tolerated, and in most pain centers, it has become the adjuvant analgesic of choice in the treatment of diabetic truncal neuropathy. Gabapentin has a large therapeutic window, but the physician is cautioned to start at the low end of the dosage spectrum and titrate upward slowly to avoid central nervous system side effects, including sedation and fatigue. The following recommended dosage schedule can minimize side effects and encourage compliance: a single bedtime dose of 300 mg for 2 nights followed by 300 mg twice a day for an additional 2 days. If the patient is tolerating this twice-daily dosing, the dosage may be increased to 300 mg three times a day. Most patients begin to experience pain relief at this dosage. Additional titration upward can be carried out in 300-mg increments as side effects allow. A total greater than 3600 mg/day in divided doses is not currently recommended. The use of 600- or 800-mg tablets can simplify maintenance dosing after titration has been completed.

Pregabalin represents a reasonable alternative to gabapentin and is better tolerated in some patients. Pregabalin is started at 50 mg three times a day and may be titrated upward to 100 mg three times a day as side effects allow. Because pregabalin is excreted primarily by the kidneys, the dosage should be decreased in patients with compromised renal function.

Antiarrhythmics

Mexiletine is an antiarrhythmic drug that may be effective in the management of diabetic truncal neuropathy. Some pain specialists believe that mexiletine is especially useful in patients with primarily sharp, lancinating pain or burning pain. Unfortunately, this drug is poorly tolerated by most patients and should be reserved for those who do not respond to first-line pharmacologic treatments such as gabapentin or nortriptyline alone or in combination with neural blockade.

Topical agents

Some clinicians have reported the successful treatment of diabetic truncal neuropathy with topical application of capsaicin. An extract of chili peppers, capsaicin is thought to relieve neuropathic pain by depleting substance P. The side effects of capsaicin include significant burning and erythema, however, and thus limit its use.

Topical lidocaine administered by transdermal patch or in a gel can also provide short-term relief of the pain of diabetic truncal neuropathy. This drug should be used with caution in patients taking mexiletine because of the potential for cumulative local anesthetic toxicity. Whether topical lidocaine has a role in the long-term treatment of diabetic truncal neuropathy remains to be seen.

Analgesics

In general, neuropathic pain responds poorly to analgesic compounds. The simple analgesics, including acetaminophen and aspirin, can be used in combination with antidepressants and anticonvulsants, but care must be taken not to exceed the recommended daily dose because renal or hepatic side effects may occur. The nonsteroidal antiinflammatory drugs may also provide a modicum of pain relief when they are used with antidepressants and anticonvulsants. Because of the nephrotoxicity of this class of drugs, however, they should be used with extreme caution in diabetic patients, given the high incidence of diabetic nephropathy, even early in the course of the disease. The role of cyclooxygenase-2 inhibitors in the palliation of the pain of diabetic truncal neuropathy has not been adequately studied.

The pain of diabetic truncal neuropathy responds poorly to treatment with opioid analgesics. Given the significant central nervous system and gastrointestinal side effects, coupled with the problems of tolerance, dependence, and addiction, opioid analgesics should rarely, if ever, be used as a primary treatment for the pain of diabetic truncal neuropathy. If an opioid analgesic is being considered, however, tramadol may be a reasonable choice; it binds weakly to the opioid receptors and may provide some symptomatic relief. Tramadol should be used with care in combination with antidepressants to avoid the increased risk of seizures.

Cannabinoids

Considerable anecdotal evidence and advocacy support a possible beneficial role for cannabinoids in the treatment of diabetic peripheral neuropathy. Large-scale trials are under way to determine if cannabinoids offer advantages over other traditional treatments for this debilitating condition.

Neural blockade

Neural blockade with local anesthetic alone or in combination with steroid can be useful in the management of both acute and chronic pain associated with diabetic truncal neuropathy. Thoracic epidural or intercostal nerve block with local anesthetic, steroid, or both may be beneficial (Fig. 10.7). Occasionally, neuroaugmentation by spinal cord stimulation may provide significant pain relief in patients who have not been helped by more conservative measures. Neurodestructive procedures are rarely, if ever, indicated to treat the pain of diabetic truncal neuropathy. They often worsen the patient's pain and cause functional disability.

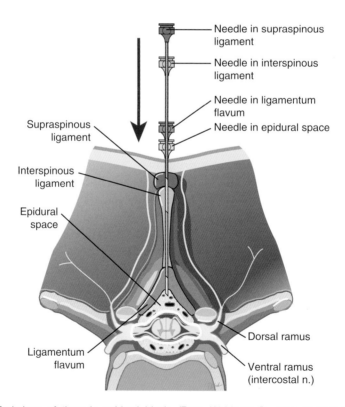

Fig. 10.7 Technique of thoracic epidural block. (From Waldman S. *Atlas of Interventional Pain Management*. ed. 5. Philadelphia: Elsevier; 2021 [Fig. 65-4].)

HIGH-YIELD TAKEAWAYS

- The patient is afebrile, making an acute infectious etiology unlikely.
- The patient's symptomatology is thought to be the result of a well-known complication of poorly controlled diabetes and diabetic truncal neuropathy.
- Physical examination and testing should focus on identification of the pathologic processes that may mimic the clinical presentation of diabetic truncal neuropathy.
- The patient exhibits neurologic and physical examination findings that are highly suggestive of diabetic truncal neuropathy.
- The patient has significant complications related to diabetes mellitus, including diabetic retinopathy and nephropathy.
- The patient's markedly elevated HbA1c level suggests long-standing poor glycemic control.
- EMG and nerve conduction velocity testing will help delineate the location and degree of nerve compromise in patients suffering from diabetic neuropathy.

Suggested Readings

Janahi NM, Santos D, Blyth C, et al. Diabetic peripheral neuropathy, is it an autoimmune disease? *Immunol Lett*. 2015;168(1):73–79.

Otto-Buczkowska E, Dryżałowski M. Neuropathy in young diabetic patients. *Pediatr Pol*. 2016;91(2):142–148.

Selvarajah D, Gandhi R, Tesfaye S. Cannabinoids and their effects on painful neuropathy. In: Preedy VR. *Handbook of Cannabis and Related Pathologies*. ed. 1. San Diego: Academic Press; 2017:905–916.

Sloan G, Shillo P, Selvarajah D, et al. A new look at painful diabetic neuropathy. *Diabetes Res Clin Pract*. 2018;144:177–191.

Waldman SD. Diabetic truncal neuropathy. In: *Atlas of Common Pain Syndromes*. ed. 4. Philadelphia: Elsevier; 2019:250–253.

Waldman SD. Intercostal nerve block. In: *Pain Review*. ed. 2. Philadelphia: Elsevier; 2017:454–455.

Waldman SD. Thoracic epidural block: midline approach. In: *Atlas of Interventional Pain Management*. ed. 5. Philadelphia: Saunders; 2021:328–338.

Chuck Connors

A 72-Year-Old Male With Persistent Pain Following a Thoracotomy for Lung Cancer

- Learn the common causes of pain following thoracic surgery.
- Develop an understanding of the anatomy and innervation of the chest wall and thorax.
- Develop an understanding of the unique relationship of the intercostal nerve to the rib.
- Develop an understanding of the causes of postthoracotomy pain.
- Develop an understanding of the differential diagnosis of postthoracotomy pain.
- Learn the clinical presentation of postthoracotomy pain.
- Learn how to use physical examination to postthoracotomy pain.
- Develop an understanding of the treatment options for postthoracotomy pain.

Chuck Connors

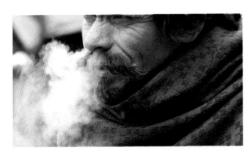

My first thought when I entered the exam room was that something was on fire. It took me a couple of beats to realize that it was Chuck, who smelled like a pile of smoldering newspapers. So much for my stop smoking lecture. Chuck Connors is a 72-year-old retired shop teacher with the chief complaint of, "Ever since I had my lung cancer surgery, my incision has been killing me." Chuck stated that he wished he had never had it, as the pain since the surgery had just about done him in. "Doctor, I am convinced that surgeon cut something she shouldn't have. She said they got it all, but if I had known that I was going to have to sleep in a chair, I would have said no to going under the knife! I must be the biggest idiot in the world. I'm an old man! I should have known better." I tried to convince Chuck that he had done the right thing, but I could tell that he wasn't going to change his mind in this regard when I saw the truculent look on his face. "Still smoking?" I asked. "Doctor, it's all I have left. Please don't start in again. Get rid of the pain, and then you can yell at me. Until then, please change the subject to how you are going to relieve this pain."

Chuck said that he didn't remember much about the surgery, but he clearly remembers waking up with a sharp pain in his side that was like a shock running from his surgical wound into the front of his chest. He said his chest incision still hurt a bit, but it was this electric shocklike pain that was the issue at hand. "Doctor, It's 24/7! I can't sleep in bed because every time I move I get the shock, and it wakes me up. Ever try sleeping in a chair every night? Take it from me, it is not much fun." Chuck said when he went for his postoperative check and talked the surgeon, she seemed disinterested and told him not to worry, that it was just a little nerve irritation from the surgery and it would get better with time, but it never did. Chuck shook his head slowly and said, "I was never so angry at a doctor. She just blew me off. You know the deal, the surgery was great, so it must be the patient's fault. She never sat down to listen to me. She was walking out the door as she blew me off. Well, I got even. Take a look at her Yelp reviews. No more five stars for her, for all the good it will do me. I tried to ask if she thought the cancer was back, but she was already out the door."

I asked Chuck if he had experienced any numbness or weakness in the area of the pain, and he replied, "Doc, it's funny that you asked because the area in front of the scar is really sensitive and feels like it's dead, just not a part of me. There is an area at about the middle of the scar that is a no-man's land. If I touch it, I cause that shock to shoot out." I asked Chuck what he had tried to make it better. He said that the pain pills they gave him after his cancer surgery just made him sick to his stomach, so he quit taking them. He said that a heating pad and a highball or two or three helped him sleep for a bit.

He also volunteered that he had quit sleeping with his pajama top on because the skin over the painful area was so sensitive, kind of like a burn or something.

I asked Chuck to show me where the pain was located, and he pointed to his left anterior chest in front of his thoracotomy scar. I asked Chuck about any fever, chills, or other constitutional symptoms such as weight loss or night sweats, and he shook his head no. He replied, "In spite of everything, I am breathing pretty well, and my appetite is good. I was never a picky eater. Give me a can of chili or chicken noodle soup and I am good to go."

On physical examination, Chuck was afebrile. His respirations were 18, his pulse was 74 and regular, and his blood pressure was 122/78. His oxygen saturation on room air was 94. Chuck's head, eyes, ears, nose, throat (HEENT) exam was normal, as was his thyroid exam. (Honestly, he smelled so strongly of tobacco smoke that it was hard to examine him. It's hard to believe that there was a time when almost everybody smoked.) Auscultation of his carotids revealed no bruits, and the pulses in all four extremities were normal. He had a regular rhythm without abnormal beats. His cardiac exam was otherwise unremarkable. There was a well-healed left thoracotomy scar without obvious defect or evidence of infection (Fig. 11.1). The minute I tried to palpate the scar, Chuck pulled back and said, "Easy, Doc. It's still kind of sore." I promised to be gentle, and about midway along the scar as I worked from posterior to anterior, I found a trigger area, and Chuck cried out in pain. "I told you to be careful, Doc! That's the spot that sends the electric shock out just to remind me I'm alive. It really hurts." The area just in front of the anterior extent of the incision was allodynic, and there was decreased sensation as I followed the dermatome anteriorly. His abdominal examination revealed no abnormal mass or organomegaly. There was no peripheral edema. His low back examination was unremarkable. There was no costovertebral angle (CVA) tenderness. Visual inspection of the right chest wall was unremarkable. A careful neurologic examination was unremarkable. His prostate was slightly enlarged, but I couldn't feel any nodules. The remainder of his rectal examination was normal.

Key Clinical Points—What's Important and What's Not

THE HISTORY

- History of onset of right-sided chest wall pain immediately following a thoracotomy for lung cancer
- Associated numbness

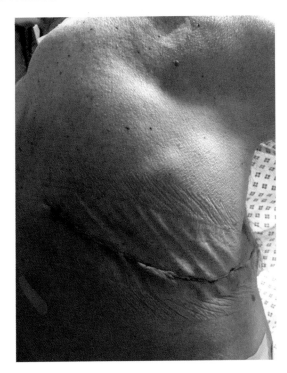

Fig. 11.1   Healing thoracotomy incision. (From Raza A, Alzetani A. Principles of posterolateral thoracotomy and pneumonectomy. *Surgery (Oxford).* 2014;32(5):266–271 [Fig. 1]. ISSN 0263-9319, https://doi.org/10.1016/j.mpsur.2014.03.001, http://www.sciencedirect.com/science/article/pii/S0263931914000593.)

- Difficulty sleeping
- Pain with electric shocklike quality in front of incision that feels like a burn
- No fever or chills

THE PHYSICAL EXAMINATION

- Patient is afebrile
- Thoracotomy scar is well healed without evidence of defect or infection (see Fig. 11.1)
- Trigger area about midscar elicits electric shocklike pain
- Area of allodynia in front of the thoracotomy scar
- Area of numbness just below the front of the scar

OTHER FINDINGS OF NOTE

- Normal HEENT examination
- Normal cardiovascular examination

- Normal pulmonary examination
- Normal abdominal examination
- No peripheral edema
- No carotid bruits

 ## What Tests Would You Like to Order?

The following tests were ordered:
- Chest x-ray
- Computed tomography (CT) scan of the thorax
- Electromyography (EMG) and nerve conduction velocity testing of the affected thoracic nerve

TEST RESULTS

The chest x-ray revealed evidence of a left thoracotomy and a smoothly margin-ated opacity at the lateral margin of the chest wall that is worrisome for malig-nancy (Fig. 11.2A).

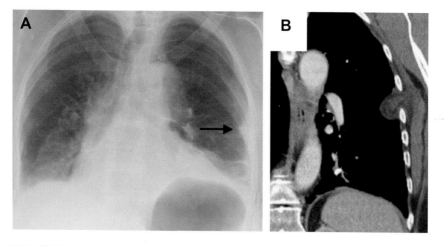

Fig. 11.2 (A) Frontal chest radiograph demonstrates a smoothly marginated opacity at the lateral mar-gin of the left midlung *(arrow)*, initially worrisome for a pleural mass such as metastasis. (B) Corresponding coronal computed tomography image illustrates herniation of fat and soft tissue through the chest wall into the extrapleural space at a level corresponding to prior surgery. (From Alpert JB, Godoy MCB, DeGroot PM, et al. Imaging the post-thoracotomy patient: anatomic changes and postoperative complications. *Radiol Clin N Am*. 2014;52(1):85–103 [Fig. 15]. ISSN 0033-8389, ISBN 9780323264105, https://doi.org/10.1016/j.rcl.2013.08.008, http://www.sciencedirect.com/science/article/pii/S0033838913001474.)

Coronal CT revealed a herniation of fat and soft tissue through the chest wall into the extrapleural space at the site of the previous thoracotomy (see Fig. 11.2B).

EMG and nerve conduction velocity testing revealed denervation of the T6 dermatome on the left.

 ## Clinical Correlation—Putting It All Together

What is the diagnosis?
- Postthoracotomy pain

The Science Behind the Diagnosis

ANATOMY

Exiting their respective intervertebral foramen and passing just below the transverse process are the spinal nerves. After exiting the intervertebral foramen, the spinal nerve gives off a recurrent branch that loops back through the foramen to provide innervation to the spinal ligaments, meninges, and its respective vertebra. It can be an important contributor to spinal pain. The spinal nerve also provides fibers to the sympathetic nervous system and the thoracic sympathetic chain via the myelinated preganglionic fibers of the white rami communicantes as well as the unmyelinated postganglionic fibers of the gray rami communicantes (Fig. 11.3). The spinal nerve then separates into a posterior and an anterior primary division. The posterior division courses posteriorly and along with its branches, provides innervation to the facet joints and the muscles and skin of the back (see Fig. 11.3). The larger anterior division gives off the intercostal nerve, which courses laterally to pass into the subcostal groove beneath the rib along with the intercostal vein and artery to become the respective intercostal nerves (Fig. 11.4). The 12th thoracic nerve courses beneath the 12th rib and is called the subcostal nerve. It is unique in that it gives off a branch to the first lumbar nerve, thus contributing to the lumbar plexus. The intercostal and subcostal nerves provide the innervation to the skin, muscles, ribs, and parietal pleura and parietal peritoneum.

CLINICAL SYNDROME

Essentially, all patients who undergo thoracotomy suffer from acute postoperative pain. This acute pain syndrome invariably responds to the rational use of systemic and spinal opioids, as well as intercostal nerve block. Unfortunately, in a few patients who undergo thoracotomy, the pain persists beyond the postoperative period and can be difficult to treat. The causes of postthoracotomy pain

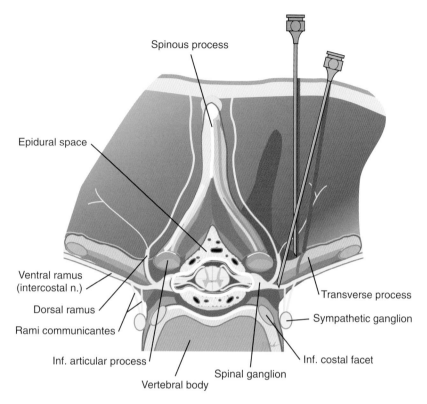

Fig. 11.3 The anatomy of the thoracic spinal nerve as it exits the intervertebral foramen. (From Waldman S. *Atlas of Interventional Pain Management*. ed. 5. Philadelphia: Elsevier; 2021 [Fig. 68.7].)

syndrome are listed in Box 11.1 and include direct surgical trauma, fractured ribs, compressive neuropathy, neuroma, and stretch injuries. When the syndrome is caused by fractured ribs, it produces local pain that is worse with deep inspiration, coughing, or movement of the affected ribs. The other causes of the syndrome result in moderate to severe pain that is constant and follows the distribution of the affected intercostal nerves. The pain may be characterized as neuritic and may occasionally have a dysesthetic quality.

SIGNS AND SYMPTOMS

Physical examination generally reveals tenderness along the healed thoracotomy incision. Occasionally, palpation of the scar elicits paresthesias, a finding suggestive of neuroma formation. Patients suffering from postthoracotomy syndrome may attempt to splint or protect the affected area. Careful sensory examination of the affected dermatomes may reveal decreased sensation or allodynia. With significant motor involvement of the subcostal nerve, patients may complain

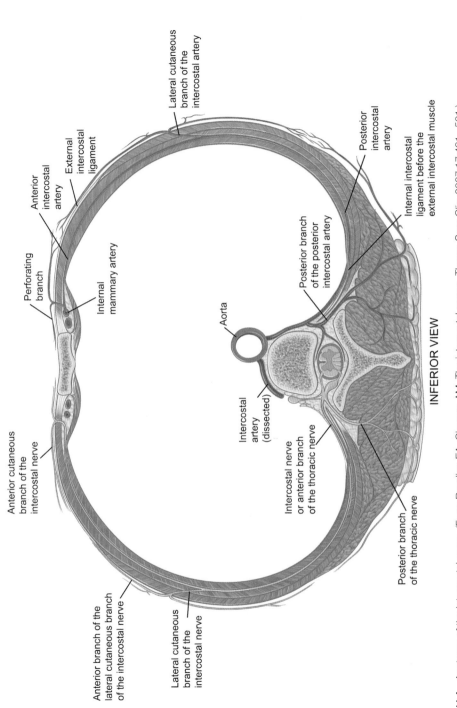

Anterior cutaneous
branch of the
intercostal nerve

Perforating
branch

Internal
mammary artery

Anterior
intercostal
artery

External
intercostal
ligament

Lateral cutaneous
branch of the
intercostal artery

Posterior
intercostal
artery

Internal intercostal
ligament before the
external intercostal muscle

Posterior branch
of the posterior
intercostal artery

Aorta

Intercostal
artery
(dissected)

Intercostal nerve
or anterior branch
of the thoracic nerve

Posterior branch
of the thoracic nerve

Lateral cutaneous
branch of the
intercostal nerve

Anterior branch of the
lateral cutaneous branch
of the intercostal nerve

INFERIOR VIEW

Fig. 11.4 Anatomy of the intercostal nerve. (From Rendina EA, Ciccone AM. The intercostal space. *Thorac Surg Clin.* 2007;17:491–501.)

BOX 11.1 ■ Causes of Postthoracotomy Pain Syndrome

Direct surgical trauma to the intercostal nerves
Fractured ribs resulting from use of the rib spreader
Compressive neuropathy of the intercostal nerves resulting from direct compression by
  retractors
Cutaneous neuroma formation
Stretch injuries to the intercostal nerves at the costovertebral junction

---

BOX 11.2 ■ Complications Following Thoracotomy

Early postoperative complications
  Pulmonary edema
  Acute lung injury/acute respiratory distress syndrome
  Pneumonia
  Hemorrhage/hemothorax
  Chylothorax
  Dehiscence of bronchial stump, formation of bronchopleural fistula
  Esophagopleural fistula
  Empyema
  Lobar torsion
  Cardiac herniation
  Gossypiboma
Late postoperative complications
  Pneumonia
  Disease recurrence (tumor, infection)
  Dehiscence of bronchial stump, formation of bronchopleural fistula
  Esophagopleural fistula
  Empyema
  Stricture of bronchial anastomosis
  Pulmonary artery stump thrombosis
  Postpneumonectomy syndrome
  Herniation of lung or chest wall soft tissues via thoracotomy defect
  Gossypiboma

Modified from Alpert JB, Godoy MCB, DeGroot PM, et al. Imaging the post-thoracotomy patient: anatomic changes and postoperative complications. *Radiol Clin N Am.* 2014;52(1):85–103. ISSN 0033-8389, ISBN 9780323264105, https://doi.org/10.1016/j.rcl.2013.08.008, http://www.sciencedirect.com/science/article/pii/S0033838913001474.)

---

that the abdomen bulges outward. Occasionally, patients suffering from post-thoracotomy syndrome develop reflex sympathetic dystrophy of the ipsilateral upper extremity that if left untreated may result in a frozen shoulder.

TESTING

For all patients who present with postthoracotomy pain, plain radiographs of the chest are indicated to rule out occult rib fractures and other causes of post-thoracotomy pain, including infection and tumor (Box 11.2). The opacification of the hemithorax that occurs following pneumonectomy can complicate the radiographic diagnosis (Fig. 11.5). Radionuclide bone scanning may be useful to exclude occult fractures of the ribs or sternum. Based on the patient's clinical presentation, additional testing may be warranted, including a complete blood count, prostate-specific antigen level, erythrocyte sedimentation rate, and antinuclear antibody testing. CT scanning of the thoracic contents is indicated if an occult mass or pleural disease is suspected (Fig. 11.6; also see Fig. 11.2). Injection of the nerve thought to be subserving the patient's pain may serve as both a diagnostic and a therapeutic maneuver (see Fig. 11.3). EMG is useful in distinguishing injury of the distal intercostal nerve from stretch injuries of the intercostal nerve at the costovertebral junction.

DIFFERENTIAL DIAGNOSIS

The pain of postthoracotomy syndrome may be mistaken for pain of cardiac or gallbladder origin, thus leading to visits to the emergency department and unnecessary cardiac and gastrointestinal workups. In the presence of trauma, postthoracotomy syndrome may coexist with fractured ribs or fractures of the sternum itself, which can be missed on plain radiographs and may require radionuclide bone scanning for proper identification. Tietze syndrome, which is painful enlargement of the upper costochondral cartilage associated with viral infection, may be confused with postthoracotomy syndrome.

Neuropathic pain involving the chest wall may also be confused or coexist with postthoracotomy syndrome. Examples of such neuropathic pain syndromes include diabetic polyneuropathies and acute herpes zoster involving the thoracic nerves. Diseases of the structures of the mediastinum are possible and may be difficult to diagnose. Pathologic processes that inflame the pleura, such as pulmonary embolus, infection, and Bornholm disease, may also confuse the diagnosis and complicate treatment (see Fig. 11.6).

TREATMENT

Initial treatment of postthoracotomy syndrome includes a combination of simple analgesics and nonsteroidal antiinflammatory drugs or cyclooxygenase-2 inhibitors. If these medications do not adequately control the patient's symptoms, a tricyclic antidepressant or gabapentin should be added.

Traditionally, tricyclic antidepressants have been a mainstay in the palliation of pain caused by postthoracotomy syndrome. Controlled studies have demonstrated the efficacy of amitriptyline, and nortriptyline and desipramine have also proved to be clinically useful. Unfortunately, this class of drugs is associated with significant anticholinergic side effects, including dry mouth, constipation, sedation, and urinary retention. These drugs should be used with caution in

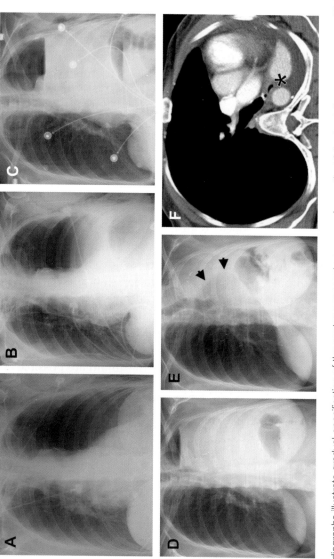

Fig. 11.5 Frontal radiographs illustrate gradual opacification of the postpneumonectomy space in a patient following left pneumonectomy. (A) Immediately after surgery, air fills the postpneumonectomy space. The trachea is in the midline, and there is slight vascular congestion in the remaining lung. Subcutaneous air is noted. (B) Radiograph on postoperative day 1 demonstrates fluid occupying one-third of the left hemithorax. The left hemidiaphragm is elevated. (C) By postoperative day 4, roughly two-thirds of the pneumonectomy space is fluid filled. (D) Three weeks after surgery, a small volume of air remains at the left apex. (E) Months later, the hemithorax is completely opacified; the heart has shifted into the left chest, and the right lung has hyperinflated (*arrowheads*). (F) Corresponding axial computed tomography images in soft tissue window confirms expected postoperative changes. Only a small volume of fluid remains in the postsurgical space. The esophagus (*asterisk*) is located adjacent to the left bronchial stump. (From Alpert JB, Godoy MCB, DeGroot PM, et al. Imaging the postthoracotomy patient: anatomic changes and postoperative complications. *Radiol Clin N Am.* 2014;52(1):85–103 [Fig. 6]. ISSN 0033-8389, ISBN 9780323264105, nttps://doi.org/10.1016/j.rcl.2013.08.008.)

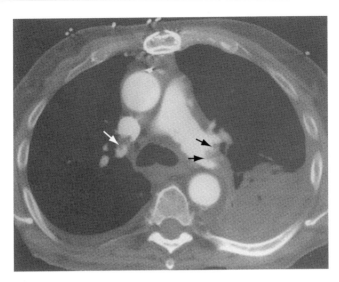

Fig. 11.6 Computed tomography demonstrates bilateral pulmonary emboli in the presence of left lower lobe consolidation and bilateral pleural effusions. A large embolus is visible in the left main pulmonary artery *(black arrows)*, and a small embolus is evident in the proximal right upper lobe pulmonary artery *(white arrow)*. (From Grainger RG, Allison DJ, Adam A, Dixon AK. *Grainger & Allison's Diagnostic Radiology: A Textbook of Medical Imaging.* ed. 4. Philadelphia: Churchill Livingstone; 2002.)

patients suffering from glaucoma, cardiac arrhythmia, and prostatism. To minimize side effects and encourage compliance, the physician should start amitriptyline or nortriptyline at a 10-mg dose at bedtime; the dose can then be titrated upward to 25 mg at bedtime as side effects allow. Subsequently, upward titration in 25-mg increments can be carried out each week as side effects allow. Even at lower doses, patients generally report a rapid reduction in sleep disturbance and begin to experience some pain relief in 10 to 14 days. If the patient does not show any reduction in pain as the dose is being titrated upward, the addition of gabapentin alone or in combination with nerve blocks is recommended. The selective serotonin reuptake inhibitors, such as fluoxetine, have also been used to treat the pain of postthoracotomy syndrome, and although these drugs are better tolerated than are the tricyclic antidepressants, they appear to be less efficacious.

If the antidepressant compounds are ineffective or contraindicated, gabapentin is a reasonable alternative. Gabapentin is started at a 300-mg dose at bedtime for 2 nights. The patient should be cautioned about potential side effects, including dizziness, sedation, confusion, and rash. The drug is then increased in 300-mg increments given in equally divided doses over 2 days as side effects allow until pain relief is obtained or a total dosage of 2400 mg/day is reached. At this point, if the patient has experienced partial pain relief, blood values are measured, and the drug is carefully titrated upward using 100-mg tablets. Rarely is a dose greater than 3600 mg/day required. Pregabalin represents a reasonable

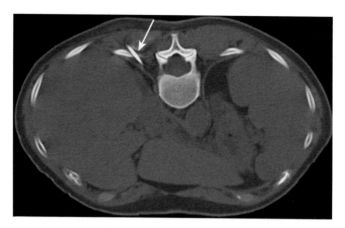

Fig. 11.7 Axial computed tomographic (CT) image of a 45-year-old woman with history of postthoracotomy pain syndrome. The interprocedural CT image shows a cryoablation probe *(arrow)* placed just inferior to the 12th right posterior rib. (From Moore W, Kolnick D, Tan J, Yu HS. CT guided percutaneous cryoneurolysis for post-thoracotomy pain syndrome: early experience and effectiveness. *Acad Radiol.* 2010;17(5):603–606.)

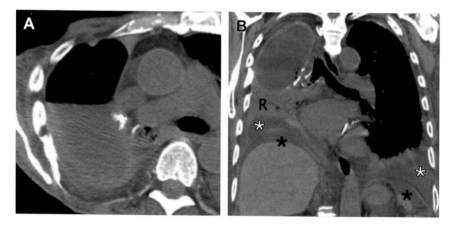

Fig. 11.8 Empyema in a 79-year-old man after right upper lobectomy. (A) Axial computed tomography (CT) image shows an air-fluid level in the superior right hemithorax with associated pleural thickening. There is high-density surgical material at the hilum, and the bronchus intermedius is filled with debris. (B) Reformatted coronal CT image illustrates empyema compressing the atelectatic right lung *(R)*. A small amount of pleural fluid *(white asterisks)* is seen at both lung bases, and there is ascites *(black asterisks)* in the upper abdomen. (From Alpert JB, Godoy MCB, DeGroot PM, et al. Imaging the post-thoracotomy patient: anatomic changes and postoperative complications. *Radiol Clin N Am.* 2014;52(1):85–103 [Fig. 9]. ISSN 0033-8389, ISBN 9780323264105, https://doi.org/10.1016/j.rcl.2013.08.008.)

alternative to gabapentin and is better tolerated in some patients. Pregabalin is started at 50 mg three times a day and may be titrated upward to 100 mg three times a day as side effects allow. Because pregabalin is excreted primarily by the kidneys, the dosage should be decreased in patients with compromised renal function. Low-dose ketamine has also been recommended as an alternative to the abovementioned medications in the management of postthoracotomy pain.

The local application of heat and cold or the use of an elastic rib belt may also provide symptomatic relief. Concurrent use of a transdermal lidocaine patch may also offer additional pain relief in patients suffering from postthoracotomy pain. For patients who do not respond to these treatment modalities, injection using local anesthetic and steroid is a reasonable next step. The use of spinal cord stimulation and neurodestructive procedures should be reserved for patients who fail to respond to more conservative measures (Fig. 11.7).

COMPLICATIONS AND PITFALLS

The major problem in the care of patients thought to be suffering from postthoracotomy syndrome is failure to identify potentially serious disorders of the thorax and upper abdomen (Fig. 11.8; see Box 11.2). A heightened index of suspicion is appropriate in patients with a diagnosis of malignancy or in whom a clear etiology of the pain cannot be ascertained.

HIGH-YIELD TAKEAWAYS

- The patient is afebrile, making an acute infectious etiology unlikely.
- The patient's symptomatology is thought to be the result of trauma to the intercostal nerve at the time of thoracotomy.
- The patient has the incidental finding of a chest wall herniation through the thoracotomy incision that may be contributing to his pain.
- Physical examination and testing should focus on the identification of other pathologic processes that may mimic the clinical diagnosis of postthoracotomy syndrome, especially in a patient with a history of lung cancer.
- The patient exhibits neurologic and physical examination findings that are highly suggestive of postthoracotomy pain.
- The patient's symptoms are unilateral.
- EMG and nerve conduction velocity testing will help delineate the location and degree of nerve compromise if nerve compromise is suspected.
- CT scan of the chest may help identify less common causes of compression of the affected nerve(s) (e.g., tumor, lipoma, or neural tumors).

Suggested Readings

Auinger D, Sandner-Kiesling A, Strießnig A, et al. Is there an impact of sex on acute postthoracotomy pain? A retrospective analysis. *Ann Thorac Surg*. 2020;109(4):1104–1111.

Moore W, Kolnick D, Tan J, et al. CT guided percutaneous cryoneurolysis for post-thoracotomy pain syndrome: early experience and effectiveness. *Acad Radiol*. 2010;17 (5):603–606.

Niraj G, Kelkar A, Kaushik V, et al. Audit of postoperative pain management after open thoracotomy and the incidence of chronic postthoracotomy pain in more than 500 patients at a tertiary center. *J Clin Anesth*. 2017;36:174–177.

Romero A, Garcia JEL, Joshi GP. The state of the art in preventing postthoracotomy pain. *Semin Thorac Cardiovasc Surg*. 2013;25(2):116–124.

Waldman SD. Postthoracotomy pain syndrome. In: *Pain Review*. ed. 2. Philadelphia: Saunders; 2017:267–268.

Waldman SD. Postthoracotomy pain syndrome. In: *Atlas of Common Pain Syndromes*. ed. 4. Philadelphia: Elsevier; 2019:264–267.

Yoshimura N, Iida H, Takenaka M, et al. Effect of postoperative administration of pre-gabalin for postthoracotomy pain: a randomized study. *J Cardiothorac Vasc Anesth*. 2015;29(6):1567–1572.

Lydia Lutz

A 24-Year-Old Bartender With
the Acute Onset of Severe
Abdominal Pain That Radiates
Through to Her Back

LEARNING OBJECTIVES

- Learn the common causes of abdominal pain.
- Develop an understanding of the unique anatomy of the pancreas.
- Develop an understanding of the causes of acute pancreatitis.
- Develop an understanding of the differential diagnosis of acute pancreatitis.
- Learn the clinical presentation of acute pancreatitis.
- Learn how to examine the abdomen.
- Learn how to use physical examination to identify acute pancreatitis.
- Learn how to use laboratory evaluation to identify acute pancreatitis.
- Develop an understanding of the treatment options for acute pancreatitis.

Lydia Lutz

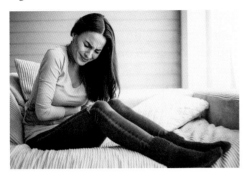

One look at Lydia and you could see that she was really sick. Lydia was always blasting in and out of the office for this and that, never anything big, sore throats, earaches, one time a Bartholin cyst. This time was different. Lydia Lutz is a 24-year-old bartender with the chief complaint of, "I feel like I'm dying." Lydia stated that over the past several days, she has had increasing upper abdominal pain that is boring through to her back. "Doctor, at first I thought I just had the 'brown bottle flu.' I hit it pretty hard last weekend. My bestie was in town, and it was nonstop fun. I thought it would go away. I took PeptoBismol and Tums, but I just got sicker and sicker. Now it's hard to lie flat in bed. I feel best when I prop myself up on the couch and hug my knees. Don't worry, Doc, I'm not pregnant. I just finished my period. This really sucks." Lydia went on to say that she would probably lose her job if she didn't get back to work within the next couple of days. I asked Lydia if she ever had anything like this before, and she said, "Now that I think about it, I've had a kind of queasy feeling in my tummy in the center up high a couple of times, but I really didn't give it much thought. I'd take some Tums and a swig of PeptoBismol and head into work. Sometimes a Brandy Alexander or two would set things right. I can make a mean Brandy Alexander. I like it with Baileys and a dash of cinnamon—it's really soothing. You should come into the bar and I'll make you one, and you'll see what I mean. It's just what the doctor ordered." With that, Lydia rolled over on her side on the exam table, moaned and pulled her knees up to her abdomen. "Doc, I am sicker than a dog. Please get me better! I feel like somebody is drilling a big hole all the way through my gut. Like they are digging to China! I think this is something more than the flu."

I asked Lydia what made the pain worse, and she said even though she didn't have much of an appetite, any time she tried to force herself to eat, she got really nauseated. She said that her stomach was really "off." She reported having diarrhea that was "really gross, really smelly." Her roommate had been giving her a hard time until she realized how sick she was. "She took off work to bring me in today. Oh, Doctor, I feel like I am going to die." As I started to examine Lydia, I began to think she was right and asked my nurse to get me a liter of lactated Ringer and an intravenous start kit. "Lydia, I think we ought to get you over to the hospital because you are pretty sick."

I asked Lydia to use one finger to point to the spot where it hurt the most, and she pointed to her epigastrium and said that it felt like someone was drilling a hole in her gut.

On physical examination, Lydia was febrile with a temperature of 100.4°F. Her respirations were 20, her pulse ox was 96 on room air, and her pulse was 92 and regular. Her blood pressure was 100/62, and she appeared acutely ill. Lydia had mild scleral icterus, which I ascertained was not good. On fundoscopic examination, her retina looked okay, and nothing else appeared abnormal about her head, eyes, ears, nose, throat (HEENT) exam, except that her breath smelled of alcohol. She was tachycardic, and I thought I could hear rales in the base of her left lung. Her thyroid was normal, and there was no adenopathy. Her abdominal examination was markedly abnormal. Even gentle palpation caused Lydia to moan. She was most tender in her epigastrium, and she was guarding her abdomen. Lydia had no localized pain with palpation of McBurney point, and there was no real rebound tenderness. Bowel sounds were markedly diminished. Visual inspection of the abdomen revealed mild distention, but I was unable to identify the presence of either the Cullen or Grey-Turner sign. There was mild costovertebral angle (CVA) tenderness. There was no peripheral edema. Her low back examination revealed some tenderness to deep palpation of the paraspinous musculature. A quick neurologic examination was normal, with no evidence of Chvostek or Trousseau sign. I asked my nurse to call an ambulance for Lydia.

Key Clinical Points—What's Important and What's Not

THE HISTORY

- Onset of severe epigastric pain that bores through to the back after a bout of heavy drinking
- Patient feels very ill
- Patient tried to manage the pain with antacids, bismuth-containing solution, and alcohol
- Patient is anorexic
- Pain is improved with flexion of the spine and bringing the knees up to the abdomen

THE PHYSICAL EXAMINATION

- Patient is febrile and tachycardic
- Patient appears acutely ill
- Patient has mild scleral icterus

- Patient is guarding the abdomen
- Diffuse tenderness in the epigastrium without rebound
- Decreased bowel sounds
- No Cullen or Grey-Turner sign identified
- Fundoscopic examination normal
- Chvostek or Trousseau sign not present

OTHER FINDINGS OF NOTE

- Tenderness to deep palpation of the lumbar paraspinous muscles
- No peripheral edema

 What Tests Would You Like to Order?

The following tests were ordered:
- Chest x-ray to identify pathology above the diaphragm responsible for the patient's symptoms as well as to identify pleural effusion
- Abdominal x-ray series with the patient in upright position to identify free air in the abdomen
- Computed tomography (CT) of the abdomen to identify occult intraabdominal pathology and to assess the severity of the acute pancreatitis
- Serum amylase
- Serum lipase
- Comprehensive metabolic profile, including liver enzymes, triglycerides, blood urea nitrogen (BUN), creatinine, and serum calcium
- Complete blood count (CBC)
- C-reactive protein as a prognostic test for the severity of acute pancreatitis
- Ultrasound of abdomen with special attention to the gallbladder

TEST RESULTS

Chest x-ray reveals a small pleural effusion on the left as evidenced by blunting of the left costophrenic angle consistent with an inflammatory process below the diaphragm (Fig. 12.1).

Abdominal x-ray series with the patient in upright position did not identify any free air in the abdomen, suggesting that a perforated viscus is not the cause of the patient's acute abdominal pain (Fig. 12.2).

CT of the abdomen revealed diffuse edema of the pancreas and moderate peripancreatic fluid consistent with acute pancreatitis (Fig. 12.3).

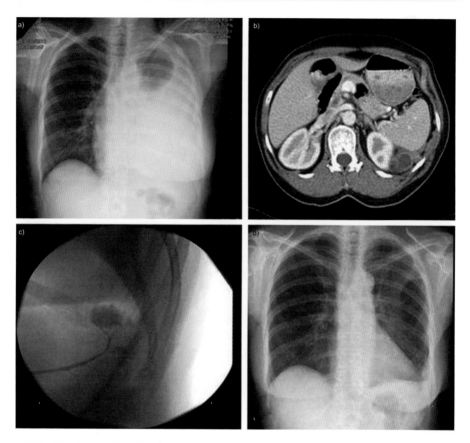

Fig. 12.1 Chest x-ray of a patient with acute pancreatitis demonstrating a small pleural effusion on the left as evidenced by blunting of the left costophrenic angle. (a–d) Radiographic imaging of acute pancreatitis.

Serum amylase was over three times normal at 265 U/L.

Serum lipase was elevated at 188 U/L.

Comprehensive metabolic profile revealed a slightly elevated aspartate aminotransferase and serum glutamic-oxaloacetic transaminase; BUN and creatinine were normal, as was serum calcium.

CBC revealed a hemoglobin of 12.4 with an elevated white count to 12,800 with a left shift.

C-reactive protein was elevated at 12, suggesting moderately severe acute pancreatitis.

Ultrasound of abdomen with special attention to the gallbladder revealed no evidence of gall bladder disease, but peripancreatic inflammation was noted (Fig. 12.4).

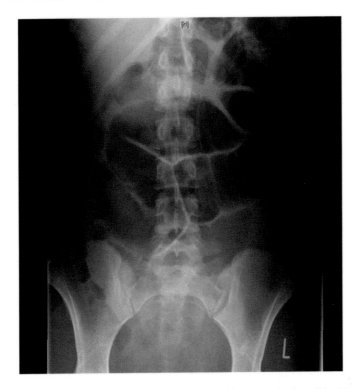

Fig. 12.2 Abdominal x-ray of a patient with acute pancreatitis demonstrating dilated loops of small bowel in the upper and midabdomen. No free air is noted.

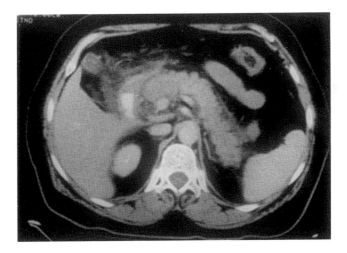

Fig. 12.3 Computed tomography scan reveals findings consistent with acute pancreatitis, including diffuse edema of the pancreas and moderate peripancreatic fluid. (From Elmas N. The role of diagnostic radiology in pancreatitis. *Eur J Radiol*. 2001;38(2):120–132 [Fig. 2]. ISSN 0720-048X, https://doi.org/10.1016/S0720-048X(01)00297-2, http://www.sciencedirect.com/science/article/pii/S0720048X01002972.)

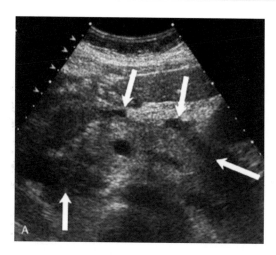

Fig. 12.4 Ultrasound of a patient with acute pancreatitis demonstrating peripancreatic inflammation as evidenced by hypoechoic inflammation ventral to the body and head and dorsal to the head *(arrows)*. (From Tchelepi H, Ralls PW. Ultrasound of acute pancreatitis. *Ultrasound Clin*. 2007;2(3):415–422 [Fig. 3]. ISSN 1556-858X, https://doi.org/10.1016/j.cult.2007.08.009, http://www.sciencedirect.com/science/article/pii/S1556858X07000746.)

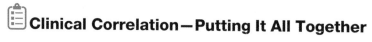 **Clinical Correlation—Putting It All Together**

What is the diagnosis?
- Acute pancreatitis

The Science Behind the Diagnosis

ANATOMY

The pancreas lies in the retroperitoneal space just behind the stomach at the level of the first lumbar vertebra (Fig. 12.5). Nestled within the C-shaped duodenum, the pancreas is both an exocrine and endocrine gland, providing important digestive and endocrine functions. The pancreas performs its digestive functions by secreting pancreatic fluids via the pancreatic duct into the duodenum via the common bile duct to aid in digestion. This fluid contains bicarbonate to help neutralize stomach acid as well as digestive enzymes to help break down fats, carbohydrates, and protein in food entering the duodenum from the stomach. As an endocrine gland, the pancreas is primarily responsible for the regulation of blood sugar. It accomplishes this role by secreting insulin, glucagon, somatostatin, and pancreatic polypeptide into the bloodstream.

The sympathetic innervation of the abdominal viscera originates in the anterolateral horn of the spinal cord. Preganglionic fibers from T5-T12 exit the

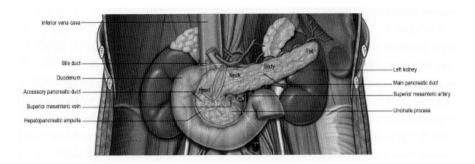

Fig. 12.5 Anatomy of the pancreas and its relationship to other adjacent anatomic structures. (From Ellis H. Anatomy of the pancreas and the spleen. *Surgery (Oxford).* 2013;31(6):263–266 [Fig. 1]. ISSN 0263-9319, https://doi.org/10.1016/j.mpsur.2013.04.001, http://www.sciencedirect.com/science/article/pii/S026393191300080X.)

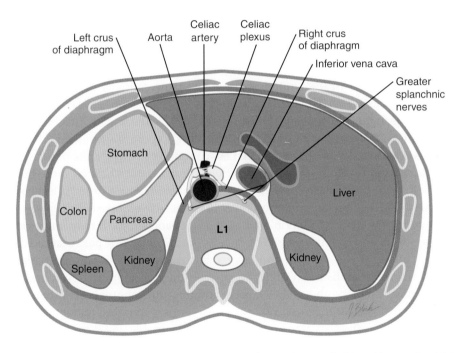

Fig. 12.6 Cross-sectional anatomy of the celiac plexus. (From Waldman S. *Atlas of Interventional Pain Management.* ed. 5. Philadelphia: Elsevier; 2021 [Fig. 84-3].)

spinal cord in conjunction with the ventral roots to join the white rami communicantes on their way to the sympathetic chain. Rather than synapsing with the sympathetic chain, these preganglionic fibers pass through it to ultimately synapse on the celiac ganglia. The greater, lesser, and least splanchnic nerves provide the major preganglionic contribution to the celiac plexus (Fig. 12.6). The greater splanchnic nerve has its origin from the T5-T10 spinal roots. The nerve travels along the thoracic paravertebral border through the crus of the diaphragm into the abdominal cavity, ending on the celiac ganglion of its respective side. The lesser splanchnic nerve arises from the T10-T11 roots and passes with the greater nerve to end at the celiac ganglion. The least splanchnic nerve arises from the T11-T12 spinal roots and passes through the diaphragm to the celiac ganglion. The celiac plexus is anterior to the crus of the diaphragm. The plexus extends in front of and around the aorta, with the greatest concentration of fibers anterior to the aorta. The relationship of the celiac plexus to the surrounding structures is as follows: The aorta lies anterior and slightly to the left of the anterior margin of the vertebral body (see Fig. 12.6). The inferior vena cava lies to the right, with the kidneys posterolateral to the great vessels. The pancreas lies anterior to the celiac plexus. All these structures lie within the retroperitoneal space.

CLINICAL SYNDROME

Acute pancreatitis is one of the most common causes of abdominal pain, with an incidence of approximately 0.5% among the general population. The mortality rate is 1% to 1.5%. In the United States, acute pancreatitis is most commonly caused by excessive alcohol consumption (Fig. 12.7); gallstones are the most frequent cause in most European countries (Fig. 12.8). Acute pancreatitis has many other causes, however, including viral infection, hypertriglyceridemia, tumor, and medications (Boxes 12.1 and 12.2). Less common causes of acute pancreatitis include scorpion venom (particularly *Tityus trinitatis*, the Trinidad large-tailed scorpion, with particularly potent venom), cardiac bypass—induced ischemia, pregnancy, cystic fibrosis, and infection with Chinese liver fluke (Fig. 12.9).

Abdominal pain is a common feature of acute pancreatitis. It may range from mild to severe and is characterized by steady, boring epigastric pain that radiates to the flanks and chest. The pain is worse in the supine position, and patients with acute pancreatitis often prefer to sit with the dorsal spine flexed and the knees drawn up to the abdomen. Nausea, vomiting, and anorexia are other common features. The pathogenesis of acute pancreatitis is complex, making the clinical presentation and sequalae of the disease quite variable (Fig. 12.10).

SIGNS AND SYMPTOMS

Patients with acute pancreatitis appear ill and anxious. Tachycardia and hypotension resulting from hypovolemia are common, as is low-grade fever. Saponification of subcutaneous fat is seen in approximately 15% of patients suffering from acute pancreatitis; a similar percentage of patients experience pulmonary complications, including pleural effusion and pleuritic pain that may compromise respiration. Diffuse abdominal tenderness with peritoneal signs is

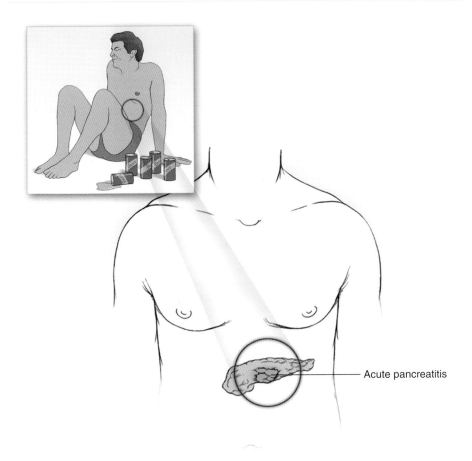

Fig. 12.7 Excessive consumption of alcohol is one of the causes of acute pancreatitis. (From Waldman S. *Atlas of Common Pain Syndromes*. ed. 4. Philadelphia: Elsevier; 2019 [Fig. 74-1].)

invariably present. A pancreatic mass or pseudocyst secondary to pancreatic edema may be palpable. If hemorrhage occurs, periumbilical ecchymosis (Cullen sign) and flank ecchymosis (Turner sign) may be present (Fig. 12.11). Both these findings suggest severe necrotizing pancreatitis and indicate a poor prognosis. If the patient has significant hypocalcemia, Chvostek or Trousseau sign may be present (Fig. 12.12).

TESTING

Elevation of serum amylase levels is the sine qua non of acute pancreatitis. Levels tend to peak at 48 to 74 hours and then begin to drift toward normal. Serum lipase remains elevated and may correlate better with actual disease

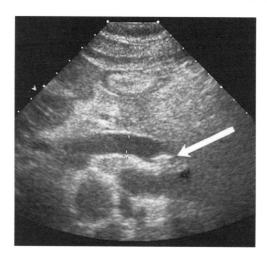

Fig. 12.8 Gallstones are the most frequent cause of acute pancreatitis in most European countries. Ultrasound image demonstrating acute a large extrahepatic bile duct stone. This oblique longitudinal sonogram of the common (extrahepatic) bile duct (calipers) shows a distal stone *(arrow)*. This duct is dilated to 12 mm. The main reason to do ultrasound in patients with acute pancreatitis is to diagnose gallstones as a cause of the disease. Finding common duct dilatation or duct stones should prompt retrograde cholangiography to remove the stone and hopefully ameliorate the clinical course of the disease. (From Tchelepi H, Ralls PW. Ultrasound of acute pancreatitis. *Ultrasound Clin.* 2007;2(3): 415–422 [Fig. 15]. ISSN 1556-858X, https://doi.org/10.1016/j.cult.2007.08.009.)

BOX 12.1 ■ Common Causes of Acute Pancreatitis

Alcohol
Gallstones
Abdominal trauma
Infections
Mumps
Viral hepatitis, cytomegalovirus
Coxsackie B virus
Ascaris
Mycoplasma pneumoniae
Medications
    Thiazide diuretics
    Furosemide
    Gliptins
    Tetracycline
    Sulfonamides
    Steroids
    Estrogens
    Azathioprine
    Pentamidine
Metabolic causes
    Hypertriglyceridemia

(Continued)

Hypercalcemia
Malnutrition
Perforating ulcers
Carcinoma of the head of the pancreas
Tumor obstructing the ampulla of Vater
Structural abnormalities
    Pancreas divisum
    Choledochocele
    Connective tissue diseases
    Postendoscopic retrograde cholangiopancreatography
Radiation induced
Hereditary causes

BOX 12.2 ■ Drugs Associated With Acute Pancreatitis

- Sulindac
- Tetracycline
- Furosemide
- Thiazide diuretics
- Chlorthaladone
- Metronidazole
- Nitrofurantoin
- Phenformin
- Procainamide
- Cancer chemotherapy drug combinations containing asparaginase
- Cisplatin
- Cimetidine
- Azothiaprine
- Steroids
- Estrogens
- Piroxicam
- Valproic acid
- Pentamidine
- Methyldopa
- Octreotide
- Didanosine
- 6-mercaptopurine
- 5-aminosalicylic acid compounds

severity. Because serum amylase levels may be elevated in other diseases, such as parotitis, amylase isozymes may be necessary to confirm a pancreatic basis for this finding. Plain radiographs of the chest are indicated for all patients who present with acute pancreatitis to identify pulmonary complications, including pleural effusion (see Fig. 12.1). Given the extrapancreatic manifestations (e.g., acute renal or hepatic failure), serial CBCs, serum calcium and glucose levels,

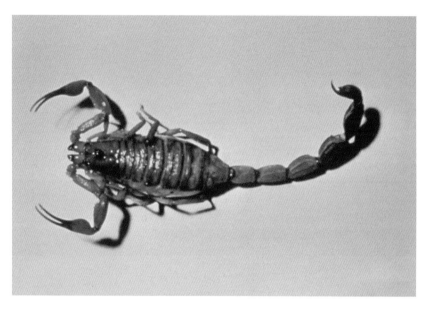

Fig. 12.9 The venom of the Trinidad scorpion *(Tityus trinitatis)* is particularly potent, as is common with small-bodied large-tailed scorpions, and can cause acute pancreatitis. (From http://www.public-domainfiles.com/show_file.php?id = 13512268819894. Retrieved May 26, 2021.)

liver function tests, and electrolytes are indicated in all patients with acute pancreatitis. There is a correlation with the degree of anion gap and the severity of acute pancreatitis. CT, ultrasound imaging, or magnetic resonance imaging of the abdomen can identify pancreatic pseudocyst and edema, and may help the clinician gauge the severity and progress of the disease (Fig. 12.13). Gallbladder evaluation with ultrasound radionuclides is indicated if gallstones may be the cause of acute pancreatitis (see Fig. 12.8). Arterial blood gas analysis can identify respiratory failure and metabolic acidosis.

DIFFERENTIAL DIAGNOSIS

The differential diagnosis includes perforated peptic ulcer, acute cholecystitis, bowel obstruction, renal calculi, myocardial infarction, mesenteric infarction, irritable bowel syndrome, diabetic ketoacidosis, and pneumonia. Rarely, the collagen vascular diseases, including systemic lupus erythematosus and polyarteritis nodosa, may mimic pancreatitis. Because the pain of acute herpes zoster may precede the rash by 3 to 5 days, it may erroneously be attributed to acute pancreatitis. Other disease that may mimic the clinical presentation of acute pancreatitis include diseases of the aorta.

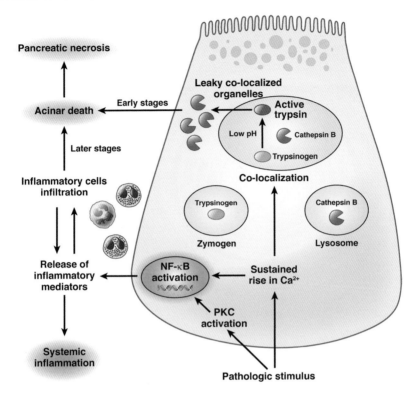

Fig. 12.10   Pathogenesis of acute pancreatitis. This paradigm demonstrates pathogenic events in acute pancreatitis. Activation of trypsinogen in the organelles formed from colocalization of lysosomal and zymogen compartments leads to leakage of cathepsin B in the cytosol, resulting in acinar death in the early stages of pancreatitis. Activation of NFκB occurs early, independent of trypsinogen activation, and leads to release of inflammatory mediators and recruitment of inflammatory cells, which causes acinar cell death in later stages of pancreatitis and drives the systemic inflammatory response seen in pancreatitis. See text for details. *PKC*, Protein kinase C. (From Saluja A, Dudeja V, Dawra R, et al. Early intraacinar events in pathogenesis of pancreatitis. *Gastroenterology.* 2019;156(7):1979–1993 [Fig. 1]. ISSN 0016-5085, https://doi.org/10.1053/j.gastro.2019.01.268, http://www.sciencedirect.com/science/article/pii/S0016508519303774.)

TREATMENT

Most cases of acute pancreatitis are self-limited and resolve within 5 to 7 days. Initial treatment is aimed primarily at allowing the pancreas to rest, which is accomplished by giving the patient nothing by mouth to decrease serum gastrin secretion and if ileus is present, by instituting nasogastric suction. Short-acting opioid analgesics such as hydrocodone are a reasonable next step if conservative measures do not control the patient's pain. If ileus is present, a parenteral opioid such as meperidine is a good alternative. Because the opioid analgesics have the potential to suppress the cough reflex and respiration, the patient must be closely

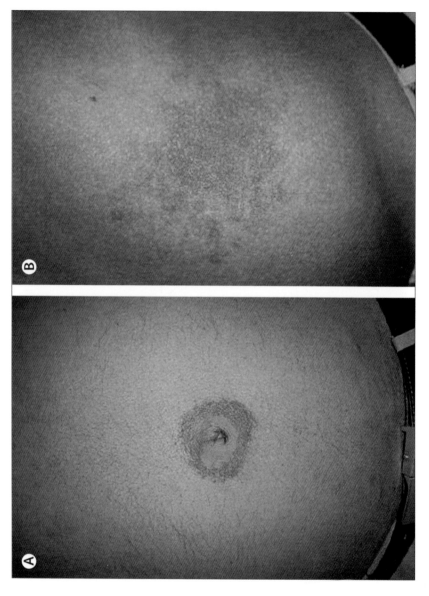

Fig. 12.11 A result of hemorrhagic pancreatitis, (A) periumbilical ecchymosis (Cullen sign) and (B) flank ecchymosis (Turner sign) may occur. (Sandeep Chauhan, Manisha Gupta, Atul Sachdev, Sanjay D'Cruz, Ikjot Kaur. Cullen's and Turner's sign associated with portal hypertension. *The Lancet.* 2008;372(9632):54. Reprinted with permission from Elsevier.)

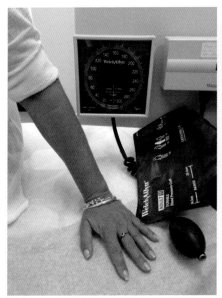
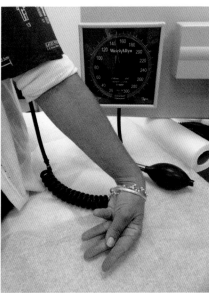

Fig. 12.12   Trousseau sign. Three minutes after inflation of the blood pressure cuff above systolic blood pressure, the patient's hand *(left panel)* shows muscular contraction *(right panel)* with flexion of the wrist, metacarpophalangeal joints, and thumb, and hyperextension of the fingers, described as "main d'accoucheur" (hand of the obstetrician). (From Bilezikian J. *The Parathyroids.* ed. 3. Waltham Academic Press; 2015 [Fig. 53-1].)

monitored and instructed in pulmonary toilet techniques. If symptoms persist, CT-guided celiac plexus block with local anesthetic and steroid is indicated and may decrease the mortality and morbidity associated with the disease (Fig. 12.14). Alternatively, continuous thoracic epidural block with local anesthetic, opioid, or both may provide adequate pain control and allow the patient to avoid the respiratory depression associated with systemic opioid analgesics.

Hypovolemia following celiac plexus block should be treated aggressively with crystalloid and colloid infusions. For prolonged cases of acute pancreatitis, parenteral nutrition is indicated to avoid malnutrition. Surgical drainage and removal of necrotic tissue may be required if severe necrotizing pancreatitis fails to respond to these treatment modalities.

COMPLICATIONS AND PITFALLS

The major pitfall when diagnosing and treating patients who are suffering from acute pancreatitis is the failure to recognize the severity of their condition and to identify and aggressively treat the extrapancreatic manifestations of acute pancreatitis. Hypovolemia, hypocalcemia, and renal and respiratory failure occur

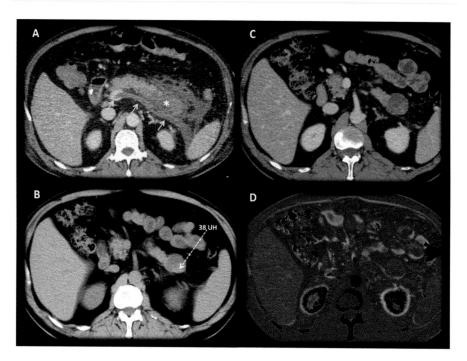

Fig. 12.13 Walled-off necrosis of the tail of the pancreas. (A) Contrast-enhanced computed tomography demonstrated with necrosis of almost 30% of the body and tail (*), yellow arrows (vascular complication with acute portal and spleen vein thrombosis); (B-D) follow-up of pancreatitis 6 months later. (B) Nonenhanced image depicts a round dense lesion in the tail of the pancreas. (C, D) Digital subtraction of the tail lesion that denotes no enhancement, representing necrotic collection with debris and avascular pseudocapsule. (From Maldonado I, Shetty A, Estay MC, et al. Acute pancreatitis imaging in MDCT: state of the art of usual and unusual local complications. 2012 Atlanta classification revisited. *Curr Prob Diagn Radiol.* 2020 [Fig. 8]. ISSN 0363-0188, https://doi.org/10.1067/j.cpradiol.2020.04.002, http://www.sciencedirect.com/science/article/pii/S0363018820300578.)

with sufficient frequency that the clinician must actively seek these potentially fatal complications and treat them aggressively.

HIGH-YIELD TAKEAWAYS

- The patient is mildly febrile.
- Physical examination and testing should focus on confirmation of the diagnosis of acute pancreatitis and to rule out other diseases that may mimic its presentation.
- The patient has boring epigastric pain that radiates to the back.
- The patient has a markedly elevated serum amylase.

(Continued)

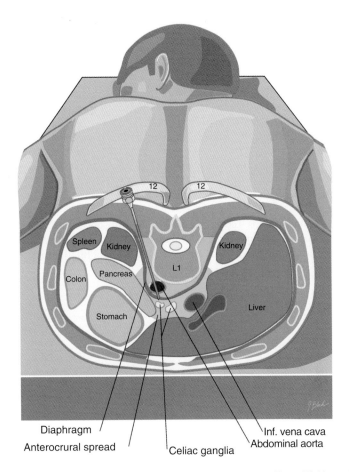

Fig. 12.14 Celiac plexus using the single-needle transaortic approach. (From Waldman SD. *Atlas of Interventional Pain Management*. ed. 2. Philadelphia: Saunders; 2004:286.)

- The patient appears acutely ill.
- Plain radiographs will provide high-yield information regarding the intrathoracic and intraabdominal contents.
- CT and ultrasound imaging will help identify the extent of the disease as well as help identify extrapancreatic complications of acute pancreatitis.

Suggested Readings

Carr RA, Rejowski BJ, Cote GA, et al. Systematic review of hypertriglyceridemia-induced acute pancreatitis: a more virulent etiology? *Pancreatology*. 2016;16(4): 469–476.

Koutroumpakis E, Slivka A, Furlan A, et al. Management and outcomes of acute pancreatitis patients over the last decade: a US tertiary-center experience. *Pancreatology*. 2017;17(1):32–40.

Mikolasevic I, Milic S, Orlic L, et al. Metabolic syndrome and acute pancreatitis. *Eur J Intern Med*. 2016;32:79–83.

Rashid N, Sharma PP, Scott RD, et al. Severe hypertriglyceridemia and factors associated with acute pancreatitis in an integrated health care system. *J Clin Lipidol*. 2016;10(4):880–890.

Waldman SD. Acute pancreatitis. In: *Atlas of Common Pain Syndromes*. ed. 4. Philadelphia: Elsevier; 2019:286–289.

Waldman SD. Acute pancreatitis. In: *Pain Review*. ed. 2. Philadelphia: Elsevier; 2017: 278–279.

Waldman SD. Celiac plexus block. In: *Pain Review*. ed. 2. Philadelphia: Elsevier; 2017: 473–476.

Waldman SD. Celiac plexus block: single-needle transaortic approach. In: *Atlas of Interventional Pain Management*. ed. 4. Philadelphia: Elsevier; 2016:401–407.

Waldman SD. The celiac plexus. In: *Pain Review*. ed. 2. Philadelphia: Elsevier; 2017: 117–118.

Brian Nguyen

A 23 Year-Old With Severe Testicular Pain and Hematuria

- Learn the common causes of testicular pain.
- Develop an understanding of the unique anatomy of the urinary tract.
- Develop an understanding of the sensory innervation of the urinary tract.
- Develop an understanding of the causes of pain associated with nephrolithiasis.
- Learn the clinical presentation of nephrolithiasis.
- Learn testing options to diagnosis nephrolithiasis.
- Learn how to use physical examination to diagnose nephrolithiasis.
- Develop an understanding of the treatment options for the various types of pain associated with nephrolithiasis.

Brian Nguyen

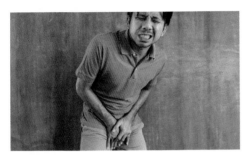

Brian Nguyen is a 23-year-old student with the chief complaint of, "Something is stabbing my left nut and I'm peeing blood." Brian stated that he was awakened from a sound sleep with the worst pain he had ever experienced. He stated that it was worse than the time he broke his leg when he tripped over a curb. "Doctor, please help me! Give me something for the pain. I can't take much more!" begged Brian. With every paroxysm of pain, Brian closed his eyes, whimpered, and paced the exam room. It was obvious he was in a lot of pain. Brian said that the pain would come out of nowhere, like someone kicked him in the nuts, and then it went away as quickly as it came. "Doctor, the pain hits and it doubles me over." Brian went on to say that he felt like he had to pee every 4 or 5 minutes, but when he tried to pee, he had to really strain to get any pee out. And when it came out, it was bloody. "Doctor, please help me. I'm afraid that I will bleed to death. Do you think I have cancer?" Brian said he felt like he needed to throw up but was afraid to because he thought it would make the pain worse. I asked, "Brian, is the pain on both sides or just on one side?" He responded, "It's always in my left nut and up by my kidney. It's never on the right." Brian went on to say that he had tried extra-strength Tylenol, but the pain just continued to get worse. I asked Brian if he ever had anything like this happen before, and he shook his head no. I asked what made it better, and he said nothing. He thought that moving around helped a little, but that nothing he has tried has really worked. Brian denied any fever or chills, but volunteered that he felt horrible.

On physical examination, Brian was afebrile. His respirations were 18, and his pulse was 88 and regular. His blood pressure was 158/88. I checked for costovertebral angle (CVA) tenderness, and when I percussed his left CVA area, Brian immediately cried out in pain and came off the exam table. He whimpered in pain and said, "Doctor, I'm begging you, warn me when you are going to do that again. It's really bad, and I need to have something to hold on to."

When I told Brian I wanted to examine his testicles, he got really upset. "Doctor, I'm begging you, please put me out before you do! I just don't know how much more of this pain I can take. It's horrible, worse than anything you can imagine. I did not know that anything could hurt this bad!" I said, "Let's start with the right testicle, Brian, and go from there. How about that?" Brian was reluctant, but said, "Do what you have to do, Doc. I have to get rid of this pain or I am done for. I am afraid of what I might do if this pain continues. I don't think I can take much more. Doctor, let me ask you something. What did I do to deserve this? I try to do good!" His right testicle exam was normal, and with great convincing, I got a quick look and feel of his left testicle, which appeared and felt completely normal. There was minimal pain with palpation. Brian was a little tender over his bladder, but I felt no abnormal mass. His fundoscopic examination was normal, as was the rest of his head, eyes, ears, nose, throat (HEENT) exam. His cardiopulmonary examination and thyroid were normal. His abdominal examination revealed no abnormal mass or organomegaly. There was no peripheral edema.

I asked Brian to point with one finger to show me where it hurt the most, and with great care to avoid touching his groin, he pointed to his left testicle. "Doctor, the pain starts way down deep in my left nut, way down deep and it shoots up into the tip of my penis." I told Brian that I was pretty sure that I knew what was going on and that we had a lot of treatment options to get on top of this pain. Brian replied, "I hope to hell you know what you are talking about, but first I really, really, really have to pee." I handed him a specimen cup. Brian limped off to the bathroom, and a few minutes later he returned and handed me his cup, which was full of blood.

Key Clinical Points—What's Important and What's Not

THE HISTORY

- No history of previous testicular pain or hematuria
- No fever or chills
- Recent onset of severe unilateral testicular pain with associated hematuria
- Urinary frequency, urgency, and stranguria
- Onset to peak of the pain is immediate
- Pain is episodic, with pain-free periods
- High degree of anxiety regarding pain and associated hematuria

THE PHYSICAL EXAMINATION

- Patient is afebrile
- Severe left CVA tenderness
- Testicular examination is normal
- Tenderness over bladder
- Urine with gross hematuria

OTHER FINDINGS OF NOTE

- Normal cardiovascular examination
- Normal pulmonary examination
- Normal abdominal examination
- No peripheral edema
- Normal neurologic examination, motor and sensory examination
- No pathologic reflexes

 ## What Tests Would You Like to Order?

The following tests were ordered:
- Dual-energy noncontrast abdominopelvic computed tomography (CT) to identify the location of the suspected kidney stone and to try and characterize its composition
- Urinalysis to identify the presence of blood, crystals, and bacteria and urinary pH (as a pH >7 suggests the presence of urea-splitting organisms such as Proteus, Pseudomonas, or Klebsiella bacteria, and/or the presence of struvite stones). A urine pH of less than 5 points the clinician toward the consideration of uric acid stones.
- Comprehensive metabolic panel, including serum creatinine and uric acid determinations, to clarify renal function and to identify the presence of hyperuricemia.
- Complete blood count (CBC) to rule out anemia of chronic disease and to identify leukocytosis associated with urosepsis.

TEST RESULTS

Dual-energy noncontrast abdominopelvic CT revealed a large stone in the left upper kidney, which was characterized as uric acid in composition (Fig. 13.1).

Urinalysis revealed gross hematuria. Uric acid crystals were also identified. No nitrates were identified on the dipstick, and the pH was 5.2.

Comprehensive metabolic panel was normal other than a markedly elevated uric acid.

CBC revealed a hemoglobin of 15.4 and a white count of 10,200 with a slight left shift.

 ## Clinical Correlation—Putting It All Together

What is the diagnosis?
- Nephrolithiasis (uric acid stone)

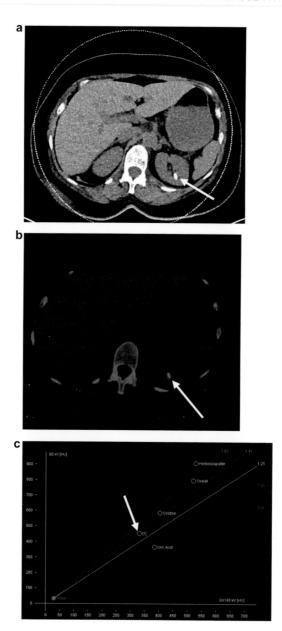

Fig. 13.1 Characterization of kidney stones using dual-energy computed tomography (DECT). Axial noncontrast CT image (a) shows a calculus at the upper pole region of left kidney. Postprocessed color map (b) shows a calcium-containing calculus in the left kidney, colored in blue. DE plot (c) confirms the composition of the stone *(arrow)* is uric acid, helping guide subsequent preventative treatment. (From McCarthy CJ, Baliyan V, Kordbacheh H, et al. Radiology of renal stone disease. *Int J Surg.* 2016;36(part D):638–646 [Fig. 4]. ISSN 1743–9191, https://doi.org/10.1016/j.ijsu.2016.10.045, http://www.sciencedirect.com/science/article/pii/S1743919116310044.)

The Science Behind the Diagnosis

ANATOMY OF THE URINARY TRACT

The upper urinary tract is comprised of the pelvicalyceal system of the kidney and the ureter (Fig. 13.2). The lower urinary tract is comprised of the bladder and urethra. The kidneys lie in the retroperitoneal space at the level of the 12th thoracic vertebra. Due to the liver, the right kidney lies slightly lower than the position of the left kidney. The ureter emerges from the hilum of the kidney and runs in a straight trajectory vertically downward within the retroperitoneal space, lying on top of the psoas major muscle. Each ureter connects its respective kidney with the urinary bladder. There are significant differences in topographic relationships of the ureter in males versus females, specifically the presence of the uterine artery in females and the vas deferens in males (Fig. 13.3).

CLINICAL CONSIDERATIONS

Nephrolithiasis, also known as renal calculi and kidney stones, is the stonelike deposit of acid salts and minerals that forms within the kidneys when these substances exist in concentrations above the saturation point within the urine. This disease occurs more commonly in males and peaks between the ages of 30 and 50 years. Nephrolithiasis occurs more commonly in Whites than in Hispanics and is much less common in Blacks. There is a family clustering of nephrolithiasis. Men have a family history of kidney stones with a two to three times greater probability of suffering from this disease.

Variables that encourage the formation of renal calculi include the presence of red blood cells, urinary casts, low calcium diets, diets high in high-fructose corn syrup and sodium, and other crystals that can form as a nucleating nidus that may promote stone formation. Ambient temperature may also correlate with the increased formation of stones, with a seasonal predilection for stone formation in the warmer southeast United States during the summer months, and in occupations exposed to high ambient temperatures (e.g., military deployments to hot desert climates). Urinary tract abnormalities such as horseshoe kidney may also increase the risk of nephrolithiasis. Some investigators believe that the obesity-metabolic syndrome-diabetes spectrum is also a risk factor for nephrolithiasis. The solubility of stone-forming solutes can also be inhibited by the presence of citrate, glycoproteins, and magnesium. The pH of the urine can increase or decrease the incidence of renal calculi, depending on which type of kidney stone is being formed, with acidic pH encouraging calcium-based stone formation.

Renal calculi are most commonly calcium based, with calcium oxalate-containing stones accounting for approximately 60% to 70% of stones (Fig. 13.4). Calcium oxalate stones are seen in patients suffering from hyperparathyroidism, malabsorption post bariatric surgery, hypervitaminosis D, diets high in

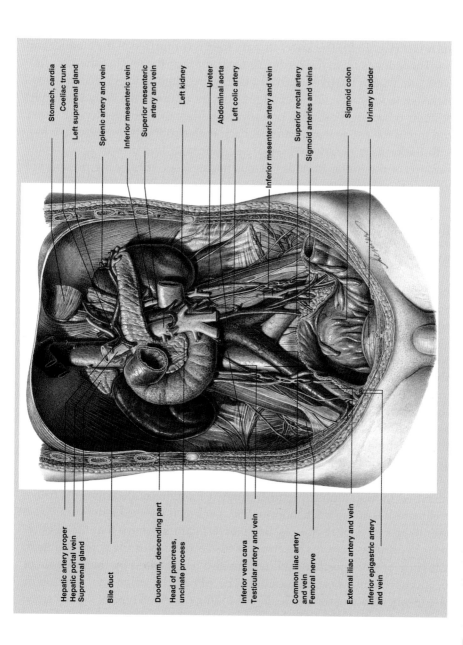

Fig. 13.2 The topographic relationships of the kidneys, ureters, and suprarenals. (From Mahadevan V. Anatomy of the kidney and ureter. *Surgery (Oxford).* 2019;37(7): 359–364 [Fig. 1]. ISSN 0263-9319, https://doi.org/10.1016/j.mpsur.2019.04.005, http://www.sciencedirect.com/science/article/pii/S0263931919300924.)

Stomach, cardia
Coeliac trunk
Left suprarenal gland

Splenic artery and vein

Inferior mesenteric vein

Superior mesenteric
artery and vein

Left kidney

Ureter
Abdominal aorta
Left colic artery

Inferior mesenteric artery and vein

Superior rectal artery
Sigmoid arteries and veins

Sigmoid colon

Urinary bladder

Hepatic artery proper
Hepatic portal vein
Suprarenal gland

Bile duct

Duodenum, descending part

Head of pancreas,
uncinate process

Inferior vena cava
Testicular artery and vein

Common iliac artery
and vein
Femoral nerve

External iliac artery and vein

Inferior epigastric artery
and vein

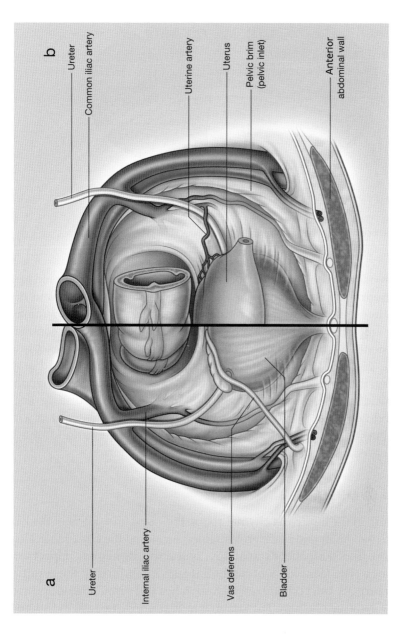

Fig. 13.3 The relationship of the intrapelvic portion of the ureter as it attaches to the bladder. Note the difference in topographic relationships of the ureter in males (a) versus females (b), specifically the location of the uterine artery in females and the vas deferens in males. (From Mahadevan V. Anatomy of the kidney and ureter. *Surgery (Oxford).* 2019;37(7):359–364. ISSN 0263-9319, https://doi.org/10.1016/j.mpsur.2019.04.005, http://www.sciencedirect.com/science/article/pii/S0263931919300924.)

a

Ureter

Internal iliac artery

Vas deferens

Bladder

b

Ureter

Common iliac artery

Uterine artery

Uterus

Pelvic brim
(pelvic inlet)

Anterior
abdominal wall

Types of kidney stones

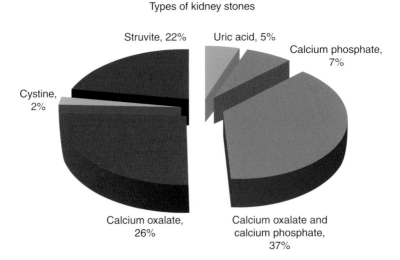

Fig. 13.4 The composition of kidney stones.

high-oxalate foods such as nuts and chocolate, and in patients with chronic pancreatitis. Calcium phosphate stones are associated with hypercalciuria and urinary alkalization secondary to renal tubular acidosis, or the use of topiramate and carbonic anhydrase inhibitors such as acetazolamide. Much less common are uric acid stones, whose formation is thought to be associated with excessive protein intake, gout, low urine output, and acidic urine. Ammonium acid urate stones and struvite stones are also less common than calcium-containing stones. Ammonium acid stones are associated with inflammatory bowel disease, laxative abuse, and ileostomy. Struvite stones are most commonly associated with urinary tract infections with urease-positive bacteria that convert urea to ammonium. Disorders of cystine transport can also cause kidney stones

SIGNS AND SYMPTOMS

Calculi can form in the intraparenchymal space, the calyx, and pelvis of the kidney, as well as the ureter and bladder. Variables, including the size of the calculus, its location, and the patient's anatomy, will affect its clinical impact and symptomatology. The symptoms of nephrolithiasis are primarily the result of increased intraurinary tract pressure, which stretches and stimulates nociceptive nerve endings in the urothelium. These pain impulses are carried via the afferent sympathetic and somatic nerves at the T11-L1 levels.

The pain of nephrolithiasis tends to wax and wane and is often colicky in nature, with spasm of the ureters and bladder occurring as stones pass distally. If the urinary obstruction is incomplete or intermittent, the pain will tend to wax

---

BOX 13.1 ■ **The Relationship of Kidney Stone Location to the Location of Perceived Pain and Associated Symptoms**

Location of Stone	Location of Pain	Associated Symptoms
Ureteropelvic junction	Severe deep flank pain, suprapubic pain	Urinary frequency/urgency, dysuria, stranguria, hematuria
Ureteral stone		
■ Upper ureter	Pain radiates to flank and lumbar areas	Intense nausea with or without vomiting, hematuria
■ Middle ureter	Pain radiates anteriorly and caudally	Intense nausea with or without vomiting, diaphoresis, hematuria
■ Distal ureter	Pain radiates into groin or testicle (men) or labia majora (women)	Intense nausea with or without vomiting, diaphoresis, hematuria
Bladder stone	Positional urinary retention, minimal to no pain	Rarely, sensation of bladder fullness, hematuria
Urethra	Severe localized pain, urinary obstruction	Deep nausea with or without vomiting, hematuria

---

and wane, with complete obstruction causing constant, severe pain. Pain may be referred to the flank, groin, testicle, or labia, with the location of the pain often reflecting the anatomic location at which the stone is obstructing the urinary system (Box 13.1). Nausea and vomiting are frequently present, as is hematuria (Fig. 13.5). Urinary urgency, frequency, dysuria, and meatal pain are also common. The patient suffering from acute kidney stones may find it difficult to find a comfortable position and may pace the floor. Fever, rigors, and chills in patients with signs and symptoms thought to be caused by kidney stones are serious findings, and immediate culture of urine and any retrieved calculi should be obtained and appropriate antibiotic therapy instituted. Anxiety and tachycardia and associated hypertension are often present.

Finding on physical examination of the patient suffering from the acute pain of nephrolithiasis includes diaphoresis, tachycardia, and hypertension. Costovertebral angle tenderness is invariably present, as is the absence of abdominal and genital findings. A commonly used diagnostic rubric to increase the specificity of diagnosis of renal calculi is the STONE score (Box 13.2). STONE is an acronym that allows easy scoring to determine the likelihood that a patient is suffering from renal and/or ureteral calculi. A score greater than 13 provides diagnostic accuracy approaching 90%.

TESTING

Unless there is significant dehydration or compromise of renal function secondary to obstruction, the serum creatinine and serum chemistry will be within normal limits, although careful attention to serum calcium levels is mandatory

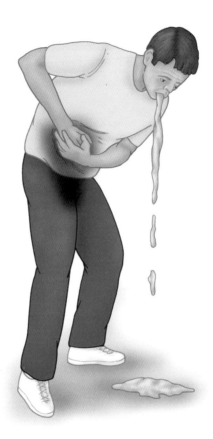

Fig. 13.5   The pain location often reflects the anatomic site at which the stone is obstructing the urinary system. Associated symptoms include nausea and vomiting, tachycardia, anxiety, and hypertension. (From Waldman S. *Atlas of Common Pain Syndromes*. ed. 4. Philadelphia: Elsevier; 2019 [Fig. 72-2].)

to help identify patients suffering from hyperparathyroidism. Leukocytosis with a left shift secondary to the stress of the pain may also be present. On urinalysis, microscopic hematuria is common, with some patients experiencing gross hematuria. Crystalluria may be observed on microscopic evaluation (Fig. 13.6). Leukouria and the presence of nitrates and leukocyte esterase in the urine is highly suggestive of a urinary tract infection. Strained urine may reveal renal calculi (Fig. 13.7).

Noncontrast, low-dose CT scans of the urinary tract have replaced intravenous pyelography as the first step in the diagnosis of nephrolithiasis (Fig. 13.8). CT scan not only provides important information as to the location and shape of the stone and the nature of obstruction but can also identify anatomic abnormalities of the urinary tract that may complicate surgical interventions (Fig. 13.9).

BOX 13.2 ■ STONE Score: A Diagnostic Rubric to Predict Nephrolithiasis

Low probability: 0–5 points
Moderate probability: 6–9 points
High probability: 10–13 points

Factor	Points
Sex	
Female	0
Male	2
Time (duration of pain)	
>24 hr	0
6–24 hr	1
<24 hr	2
Origin (race)	
Black	0
White	1
Nausea and vomiting	
None	0
Nausea alone	1
Vomiting alone	1
Both nausea and vomiting	2
Hematuria	
None	0
Present	2

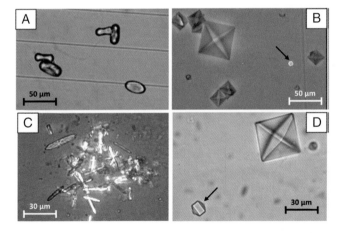

Fig. 13.6 Calcium oxalate crystals. (A) Whewellite crystals with the typical ovoid shape. (B) Typical octahedral (bipyramidal) crystals of weddellite and a small red-cell like crystal of whewellite (arrow). (C) Elongated hexagonal crystals of whewellite as found in the urine of patients after the ingestion of ethyleneglycol. (D) Octahedral and dodecahedral (arrow) crystals of weddellite. (From Frochot, V, Daudon, M, Clinical value of crystalluria and quantitative morphoconsitutional analysis of urinary calculi. *International Journal of Surgery.* Vol 36, Part D, pp. 624–632 [Fig. 1].)

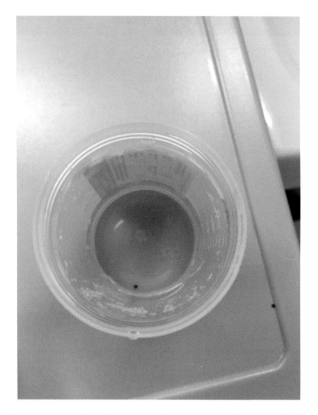

Fig. 13.7   A small renal calculus in strained urine. (From Isenberg D, Jacobs D. I just passed something in my urine. *Vis J Emerg Med*. 2016;5:31.)

Retroperitoneal ultrasound scans represent an alternative to CT scans, albeit with less sensitivity and specificity. The KUB (kidney, ureter, bladder) plain radiography or the CT scout film can also be used to follow up on the position of radiopaque stones. Dual-energy CT can be used to distinguish the composition of stones in vivo by using the difference in CT attenuation values to compare the stone's value to standard values (Fig. 13.10). Ultrasound imaging is also useful in helping to delineate the location and size of stones as well as identifying the presence of urinary obstruction (Fig. 13.11). Ultrasound has the added advantage of the avoidance of radiation.

DIFFERENTIAL DIAGNOSIS

In most patients, the diagnosis of symptomatic renal calculi is straightforward; however, basically any disorder that affects the organs that are subserved by the celiac plexus and spinal nerves T11-L2 may mimic the clinical presentation of

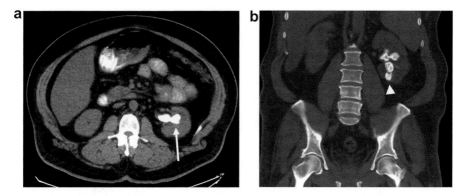

Fig. 13.8   Axial (a) and coronal (b) noncontrast computed tomography images from a patient presenting with left flank pain and gross hematuria. A large staghorn calculus *(arrow)* occupying the majority of the left renal collecting system was identified, with focal cortical scarring in the lower pole *(arrowhead)*. Volumetric analysis allows more accurate estimate of stone burden in complex calculi than morphologic measurements. (From McCarthy CJ, Baliyan V, Kordbacheh H, et al. Radiology of renal stone disease. *Int J Surg.* 2016;36(part D):638–646 [Fig. 3]. ISSN 1743-9191, https://doi.org/10.1016/j.ijsu.2016.10.045, http://www.sciencedirect.com/science/article/pii/S1743919116310044.)

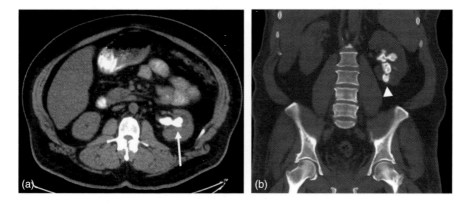

Fig. 13.9   Axial (a) and coronal (b) non-contrast CT images from a patient presenting with left flank pain and gross hematuria. A large staghorn calculus *(arrow)* occupying the majority of the left renal collecting system was identified,with focal cortical scarring in the lower pole *(arrowhead)*. Volumetric analysis allows to more accurately estimate stone burden in complex calculi than morphological measurements. (From McCarthy, C. Baliyan, V, Kordbacheh H, et al. Radiology of renal stone disease. *Int'l Journal of Surgery.* Vol 36, Part D, Dec. 2016, pp. 638–646 [Fig 3].)

kidney stones. These disorders include appendicitis, biliary colic, cholecystitis, obstructive cholelithiasis, cystitis, ileus, bowel obstruction, pyelonephritis, ovarian cyst rupture, incarcerated hernia, testicular torsion, orchitis, and viral gastroenteritis.

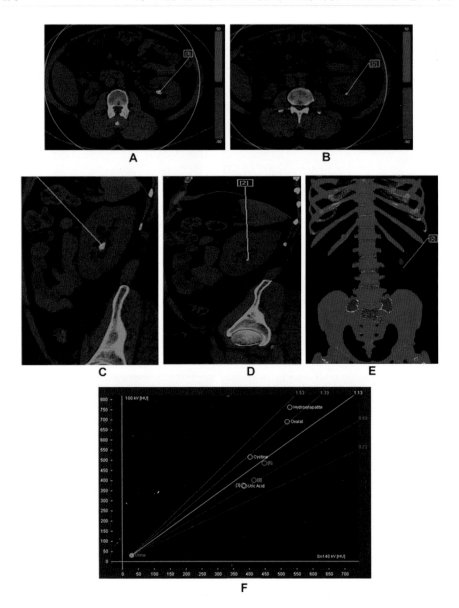

Fig. 13.10   (A—E) Axial, sagittal, and coronal color-coded dual-energy postprocessed images showing two calculi in the left middle calyx coded as red *(arrow)*, indicating uric acid calculi. (F) Graph confirming the composition of this calculus as uric acid (100/Sn140 kV ratio = 0.97). The small stone was expelled spontaneously, and chemical analysis showed that it was a uric acid stone. (From Basha MAA, AlAzzazy MZ, Enaba MM. Diagnostic validity of dual-energy CT in determination of urolithiasis chemical composition: in vivo analysis. *Egypt J Radiol Nuclear Med*. 2018;49(2):499—508 [Fig. 4]. ISSN 0378-603X, https://doi.org/10.1016/j.ejrnm.2017.12.018, http://www.sciencedirect.com/science/article/pii/S0378603X17302322.)

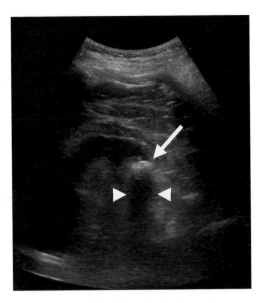

Fig. 13.11 A 79-year-old man with history of nephrolithiasis undergoing follow-up ultrasound. Sagittal image of the left kidney reveals a large stone in the lower pole *(arrow)* with posterior acoustic shadowing *(arrowheads)*. (From McCarthy CJ, Baliyan V, Kordbacheh H, et al. Radiology of renal stone disease. *Int J Surg.* 2016;36(part D):638–646 [Fig. 2]. ISSN 1743-9191, https://doi.org/10.1016/j.ijsu.2016.10.045, http://www.sciencedirect.com/science/article/pii/S17 43919116310044.)

TREATMENT

As mentioned, variables such as the size of the calculus, its location, and the patient's anatomy will affect its clinical impact and symptomatology. In general, the smaller the stone, the more likely that conservative medical treatment will be successful. With small symptomatic stones, increased fluids given orally or intravenously to increase the amount of urine may help the stone to pass and relieve the obstruction. The addition of alpha and calcium channel blockers to inhibit the contraction and peristalsis of the smooth muscle of the ureter may also help decrease symptomatology and speed stone passage.

For larger stones or in clinical situations where smaller stones fail to pass, temporizing drainage (e.g., percutaneous nephrostomy tubes), shock wave lithotripsy to fracture calculi into smaller pieces, percutaneous lithotomy, and uroendoscopic and open stone removal may be required (Fig. 13.12). Again, size and location of the offending stone(s) will dictate the best interventional therapy.

Palliation of symptoms with the use of nonopioid analgesics should be considered. Morphine and morphinelike drugs may increase intraureteral pressure

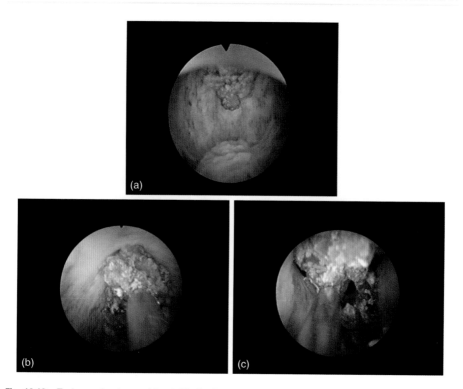

Fig. 13.12 Endoscopic stone retrieval. Urethral stone pushed retrograde into the prostatic cavity (a), fragmented at this level (b, c) to relieve urinary obstruction. (From Geavlete P. *Endoscopic Diagnosis and Treatment in Urethral Pathology.* Waltham: Academic Press; 2016 [Fig. 6−12].)

and should be avoided. Intravenous lidocaine infusions may provide palliation of the acute pain of renal and ureteral calculi. Local heat to the painful flank may also provide symptomatic relief. Thiazide diuretics may help prevent the recurrence of calcium stones, as will potassium citrate.

COMPLICATIONS AND PITFALLS

The major problem in the care of patients thought to be suffering from nephrolithiasis is related to an incorrect diagnosis in which the signs and symptoms of a life-threatening condition (e.g., dissecting aortic aneurysm) are attributed to kidney stones. A failure to promptly diagnose urosepsis associated with nephrolithiasis can cause significant mortality and morbidity. A failure to identify the underlying cause of calculi formation can result in recurrent episodes of pain and risks compromise of renal function over time.

HIGH-YIELD TAKEAWAYS

- The patient is afebrile, making an acute infectious etiology unlikely.
- The patient's pain is unilateral, and the clinical presentation is consistent with a kidney stone.
- The patient's pain is episodic, with pain-free periods between the paroxysms of pain.
- The pain has an almost instantaneous onset to peak.
- The pain is the worst the patient has ever experienced.
- The patient has significant anxiety related to the testicular pain and hematuria.
- The patient has trouble sitting still and wants to pace the room.
- Nephrolithiasis represents a true pain emergency.

Suggested Readings

Chen TT, Wang C, Ferrandino MN, et al. Radiation exposure during the evaluation and management of nephrolithiasis. *J Urol*. 2015;194(4):878—885.

Feldman HH. Rolling stones: the evaluation, prevention, and medical management of nephrolithiasis. *Physician Assist Clin*. 2016;1(1):127—147.

Ingimarsson JP, Krambeck AE, Pais Jr VM. Diagnosis and management of nephrolithiasis. *Surg Clin North Am*. 2016;96(3):517—532.

Pfau A, Knauf F. Update on nephrolithiasis: core curriculum 2016. *Am J Kidney Dis*. 2016;68(6):973—985.

Vestergaard P. Primary hyperparathyroidism and nephrolithiasis. *Ann Endocrinol (Paris)*. 2015;76(2):116—119.

Virapongse A. Nephrolithiasis. *Hosp Med Clin*. 2016;5(1):43—57.

Waldman SD. Nephrolithiasis. In: *Atlas of Common Pain Syndromes*. ed. 4. Philadelphia: Elsevier; 2019:278—281.

Vivian Zhao

A 32-Year-Old Female With Right Lower Quadrant Pain

Vivian Zhao

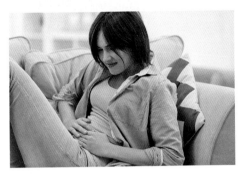

Vivian Zhao is a 32-year-old secretary with the chief complaint of, "My tummy hurts and I feel pretty crappy." Vivian noted that she woke up last night with a stomachache. She thought is must have been the spicy food she had eaten for dinner. She took some antacids, but the pain really did not get any better. Vivian went on to say that she wouldn't have bothered coming in, but the pain had changed and she really wasn't feeling any better. "Doctor, at first the pain was just a dull ache around my belly button, but as the day has progressed, it has moved down over my right ovary. I looked it up on the Internet, and I wonder if I have appendicitis. I haven't felt like eating anything, and my partner said she thought I was running a temperature. We didn't have a thermometer, and because I was feeling worse, we just decided to come on over to your office. The ride over was pretty special. Every time we hit a bump, it really hurt. When I got out of the car, it was hard to stand straight up, and walking really hurts."

I asked Vivian if anything like this has happened before. She shook her head, and said, "Absolutely not. I never get sick, but I really think that something bad is happening! Doctor, do you think I have appendicitis? Jenny, that's my partner, says it's probably just an ovarian cyst or something." Vivian denied any other gynecologic symptoms, blood in her urine, or bowel or bladder symptomatology. Her last menstrual period was about 10 days ago.

I asked Vivian if she had any change in her bowel habits over the last couple of days, and she said she was kind of constipated and now she felt like she needed to throw up. I asked Vivian to point with one finger to show me where it hurt the most. She quickly pointed to McBurney point as if she had read the textbook. I asked her if the pain radiated anywhere else, and she said not really, that over the last couple of hours, the pain seemed to have focused right on that spot.

On physical examination, Vivian was mildly febrile with a temperature of 100.8 °F. Her respirations were 18, and her pulse was 84 and regular. Her blood pressure was normal at 122/74. Her head, eyes, ears, nose, throat (HEENT) exam was normal, as was her cardiopulmonary examination. Her thyroid was normal. Her abdominal examination revealed rebound tenderness at McBurney point, as well as positive Rovsing, Blumberg, and obturator signs (Figs. 14.1 and 14.2). There was no costovertebral angle (CVA) tenderness, although percussion over the CVA exacerbated her abdominal pain.

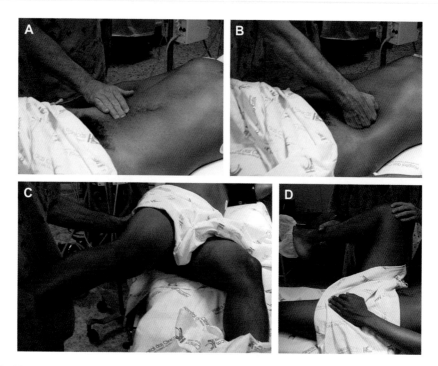

Fig. 14.1 Physical exam of a patient with right abdominal pain. (A) Blumberg sign. (B) Rovsing sign. (C) Psoas sign. (D) Obturator sign. (From Petroianu A. Diagnosis of acute appendicitis. *Int J Surg.* 2012;10(3):115–119 [Fig. 1]. ISSN 1743-9191, https://doi.org/10.1016/j.ijsu.2012.02.006, http://www. sciencedirect.com/science/article/pii/S1743919112000246.)

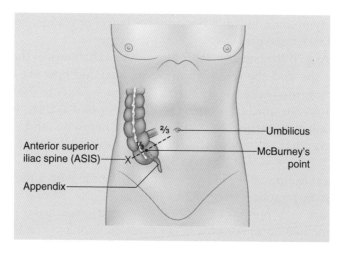

Fig. 14.2 McBurney point, the surface anatomy representing the base of the appendix. (From Sellars H, Boorman P. Acute appendicitis. *Surgery (Oxford).* 2017;35(8):432–438 [Fig. 1]. ISSN 0263-9319, https://doi.org/10.1016/j.mpsur.2017.06.002, http://www.sciencedirect.com/science/article/pii/S0263931917301345.)

There was no peripheral edema. Her low back examination was unremarkable. I did a rectal exam, which revealed tenderness on the right. Visual inspection of the abdomen was unremarkable. "Vivian," I said, "I think we are going to take a little trip to the hospital and get that appendix out." She gave me a weak smile and said, "I knew it. I need to call my mom to come be with me."

Key Clinical Points—What's Important and What's Not

THE HISTORY

- History of acute onset of periumbilical pain that migrated and localized to the right lower quadrant
- History of constipation and anorexia
- History of pain when hitting bumps while riding in the car to come to the office
- Fever was noted
- Last menstrual period 10 days ago

THE PHYSICAL EXAMINATION

- Patient is febrile
- Patient has rebound tenderness at McBurney point
- Tenderness on the right on rectal examination
- Positive Rovsing, Blumberg, and obturator tests for acute appendicitis (see Figs. 14.1 and 14.2)

OTHER FINDINGS OF NOTE

- Normal HEENT examination, decreasing the chances of mesenteric adenitis
- Normal cardiovascular examination
- Normal pulmonary examination
- No peripheral edema
- No CVA tenderness

 ## What Tests Would You Like to Order?

The following tests were ordered:
- Computed tomography (CT) scan of the abdomen
- Complete blood count
- Pregnancy test

TEST RESULTS

The CT scan of the abdomen revealed a dilated appendix with adjacent fat stranding, suggestive of mild acute appendicitis.

CBC revealed a white count of 12,400 with a shift to left.

Pregnancy test was negative.

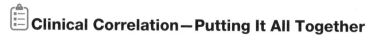

Clinical Correlation—Putting It All Together

What is the diagnosis?
- Appendicitis

The Science Behind the Diagnosis

ANATOMY

The appendix is a wormlike, pouchlike structure that is located approximately 1 inch inferior to the ileocecal valve (Fig. 14.3). It is 3 to 4 inches long and contains a lumen, which can become obstructed, causing phlegmon formation and the

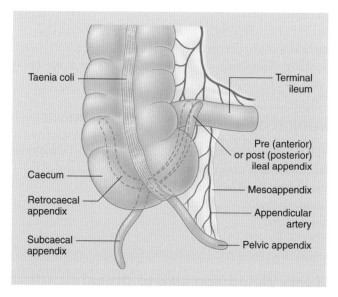

Fig. 14.3 The anatomy of the appendix. Note the mesoappendix containing the appendicular artery in its lateral edge. The dotted lines depict a number of orientations in which the appendix is found within the population (pelvic, subcaecal, retrocaecal, pre- and postileal). (From Sellars H, Boorman P. Acute appendicitis. *Surgery (Oxford)*. 2017;35(8):432–438 [Fig. 2]. ISSN 0263-9319, https://doi.org/10.1016/j. mpsur.2017.06.002, http://www.sciencedirect.com/science/article/pii/S0263931917301345.)

clinical disorder known as appendicitis. The appendix receives its blood supply from the appendicular artery, which is a branch of the ileocolic artery. Innervation of the appendix is from autonomic fibers from the ileocolic branch of the superior mesenteric plexus. The base of the anatomy is located beneath McBurney point (see Fig. 14.2).

CLINICAL PRESENTATION

Acute appendicitis is one of the most common causes of abdominal pain, with an incidence of approximately 8.5% in males and 6.7% in females. The mortality rate is approximately 0.5%. Although acute appendicitis can occur at any age, it most commonly occurs in the second or third decades. Conventional wisdom holds that acute appendicitis is the result of obstruction of the appendicular lumen, with subsequent impairment of the wall leading to perforation and phlegmon formation. More recent thinking posits that mild uncomplicated appendicitis and severe complicated appendicitis are caused by different pathologic processes and are in fact two completely separate diseases requiring very different treatments.

The diagnosis is made on clinical grounds in many countries, and appendectomy has remained the standard of care in the treatment of acute appendicitis for the last century. This is despite that approximately 15% of appendectomies yield a pathologically normal appendix and that appendectomy is not without morbidity and rarely, mortality. The routine use of imaging, including ultrasound and CT as adjuncts to the clinical diagnosis of acute appendicitis, has decreased the number of "normal result" appendectomies to approximately 10%. Recent interest in the nonsurgical management of mild uncomplicated acute appendicitis is also impacting this statistic.

Abdominal pain is a common feature of acute appendicitis (Fig. 14.4). Although the clinical presentation of the pain of acute appendicitis can be variable, its classic clinical presentation begins as mild periumbilical pain that becomes more severe and then migrates to the right lower quadrant at a point that is one-third the distance from the anterior superior iliac spine and the umbilicus, known as McBurney point (see Fig. 14.2). The pain becomes more localized and constant, with associated anorexia, nausea, vomiting, and fever. Constipation and diarrhea, as well as urinary tract symptoms, may also occur. Symptoms are usually present for less than 48 hours before the patient seeks medical attention.

SIGNS AND SYMPTOMS

Patients with acute appendicitis appear ill and anxious. A low-grade fever is often present. Patients will often flex their hips and draw up their knees in an

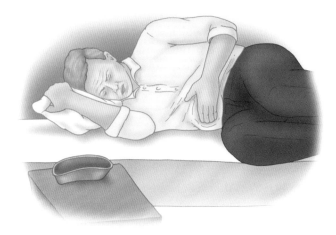

Fig. 14.4 The patient suffering from acute appendicitis will have pain localized to the right lower quadrant at McBurney point and associated anorexia, nausea, and vomiting. Low-grade fever is invariably present. (From Waldman S. *Atlas of Common Pain Syndromes*. ed. 4. Philadelphia: Elsevier; 2019 [Fig. 79-1].)

effort to splint the abdomen and decrease the pain. Early in the course of the disease, there is diffuse periumbilical tenderness and nonspecific findings, including decreased bowel sounds on physical examination. As the pain localizes to the right lower quadrant at McBurney point, peritoneal signs, including abdominal guarding, pain on percussion, and rebound tenderness, become prominent. In addition to these physical findings, a number of physical examination tests can increase the diagnostic specificity of the physical examination (Table 14.1). All exploit the consistent finding of increased pain at the point of peritoneal or structural irritation when the test is performed in patients suffering from acute appendicitis. Although nonspecific, increased right-sided pain on rectal and vaginal examination may support the diagnosis of acute appendicitis, but more importantly, it helps rule out other pathologic processes that may mimic the disease.

TESTING

Currently, there is no specific laboratory test for acute appendicitis, but the finding of leukocytosis with a left shift and elevated C-reactive protein levels increase the likelihood of acute appendicitis by a factor of 5 when history and physical findings support that clinical diagnosis. Urinalysis may reveal mild pyuria that is thought to be caused by inflammation of the ureter secondary to the proximity of the inflamed appendix to the right ureter. Recent studies

TABLE 14.1 ■ **Useful Physical Examination Tests When Diagnosing Acute Appendicitis**

Test	Maneuver	Basis of Physical Findings
McBurney point	Palpation at a point that is one-third the distance from the anterior superior iliac spine and the umbilicus yields maximal pain	Suggests peritoneal irritation at point where appendix attaches to cecum
Rovsing sign	Palpation of left lower quadrant yields pain at McBurney point	Suggests peritoneal irritation at McBurney point
Dunphy sign	Having patient cough elicits sharp pain at McBurney point	Suggests peritoneal irritation at McBurney point
Markle sign	When the standing patient drops from standing on toes to the heels with a jarring landing, the pain increases at McBurney point	Suggests peritoneal irritation at McBurney point
Obturator sign	Internal and external rotation of the flexed right hip yields pain at McBurney point	Suggests peritoneal irritation at McBurney point and may point to a retrocecal appendix
Psoas sign	Extension of the right hip or with flexion of the right hip against resistance yields pain at McBurney point	Suggests that appendix may lie against the psoas muscle
Blumberg sign	The abdomen is palpated and the pressure is suddenly released, eliciting pain	Suggests peritoneal irritation

suggest that levels of urinary 5-hydroxyindoleacetic acid (5-HIAA) may be elevated in the early stages of acute appendicitis secondary to the inflammation of serotonin-containing cells within the appendix. A downward trajectory of urinary 5-HIAA levels after initial elevations is thought to correlate with disease progression. It should be noted that pregnancy testing is mandatory in all female patients of child bearing age who present with abdominal pain.

Because of the desire to avoid unnecessary appendectomy, a scoring tool to improve the accuracy of diagnosis of acute appendicitis has been developed. The Alvarado score provides a consistent and reproducible tool to help diagnose acute appendicitis. The score is based on the ranking of symptoms and the physical and laboratory findings (Table 14.2). A score of 9 to 10 suggests that a diagnosis of appendicitis is highly probable, a score of 7 to 8 that the diagnosis is probable, and a score of 5 to 6 that the diagnosis is compatible with acute appendicitis. Experience with use of the Alvarado score suggests that appendectomy should be considered in those patients with clinical findings suggesting acute appendicitis who have an Alvarado score of 7 or greater. Other scoring systems designed to improve the accuracy of acute appendicitis have been proposed. The Andersson Inflammatory Response Score expands the parameters of the Alvarado scoring system by adding gradations of physical findings and

TABLE 14.2 ■ The Alvarado Scoring System for Acute Appendicitis

Symptoms	Migratory right iliac fossa pain	1	
	Nausea/vomiting	1	
	Anorexia	1	
Signs	Right iliac fossa tenderness	2	
	Elevation of temperature	1	
	Rebound tenderness, right iliac fossa	1	
Laboratory	Leukocytosis	2	
	Left shift	1	
Total Score	1–10		
Sum	0–4		Not likely appendicitis
	5–6		Equivocal
	7–8		Probably appendicitis
	9–10		Highly likely appendicitis

TABLE 14.3 ■ The Andersson Scoring System for Acute Appendicitis

		Andersson Inflammatory Response Score
Vomiting		1
Pain in right inferior fossa		1
Rebound tenderness or	Light	1
muscular defense	Medium	2
	Strong	3
Body temperature >38°C		0
		1
White blood cell count	10.0–14.9 × 109/L	1
	15.0 × 109/L	2
Polymorphonuclear	70%–84%	1
leukocytes	>85%	2
C-reactive protein	10–49 g/L	1
concentration	>50 g/L	2
Total score		0–12
If the sum is:		
0–4	Low probability. Outpatient follow-up if unaltered general condition.	
5–8	Indeterminate group. In-hospital active observation with rescoring/imaging or diagnostic laparoscopy, according to local traditions.	
9–12	High probability. Surgical exploration is proposed.	

laboratory parameters, including the C-reactive protein, and deducting points for temperatures above 38°C (Table 14.3).

The use of point-of-care ultrasound imaging has become a mainstay in the diagnosis of acute appendicitis. In health, appendicitis is not easily identifiable on ultrasound imaging (Fig. 14.5). As the appendix becomes inflamed, it is more

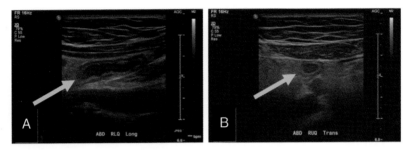

Fig. 14.5 Ultrasound demonstrating acute appendicitis. (A) Ultrasound right lower quadrant. Patient presented with a 72-hour history of abdominal pain that now localizes to the right lower quadrant. (B) Ultrasound demonstrated acute wall thickening and dilation up to 9.1 mm. Note fluid surrounding the appendix. (Green arrows) (From Murphy EEK, Berman L. Clinical evaluation of acute appendicitis. *Clin Pediatr Emerg Med.* 2014;15(3):223–230.)

easily identifiable as a noncompressible tubular structure of 7 to 9 mm in diameter that is surrounded by fluid and that lacks peristalsis. Presence of an appendicolith, phlegmon, and free air may also be identified on ultrasound imaging of the right lower quadrant. Ultrasound imaging may also provide information regarding surrounding structures or provide alternative causes for the patient's abdominal pain, especially in females of child bearing age. Limitations on the use of ultrasound to diagnose acute appendicitis include operator experience, equipment quality, the presence of large quantities of intestinal gas, patient obesity, and abnormal positioning of the appendix (e.g., retrocecal) (see Fig. 14.3).

CT has an even higher degree of specificity and sensitivity when used in the diagnosis of acute appendicitis, with a positive predictive value approaching 98%. CT can provide all of the diagnostic information obtainable on ultrasound imaging of the appendix and can accurately identify circumferential appendiceal wall thickening, periappendicular fat stranding, and adjacent adenopathy that strengthens the diagnosis of acute appendicitis (Figs. 14.6 and 14.7). Limitations on the use of CT to diagnose acute appendicitis include availability, cost, and radiation exposure, especially in children and pregnant women.

Although plain radiography of the abdomen and barium enemas were once commonly used when attempting to diagnosis acute appendicitis, their use has been supplanted by ultrasound and CT. Radionuclide scanning with technetium Tc99 labeled white cells can accurately identify acute appendicitis, but the prolonged scan times of over 4 hours and cost limit clinical utility in this setting (see Fig. 14.7). Magnetic resonance imaging has recently gained acceptance as an alternative to CT in selected patient populations, specifically, children and pregnant women who present with abdominal pain thought to be compatible with acute appendicitis, in patients whose ultrasound findings are nondiagnostic, and when patients have increased risk factors that weigh

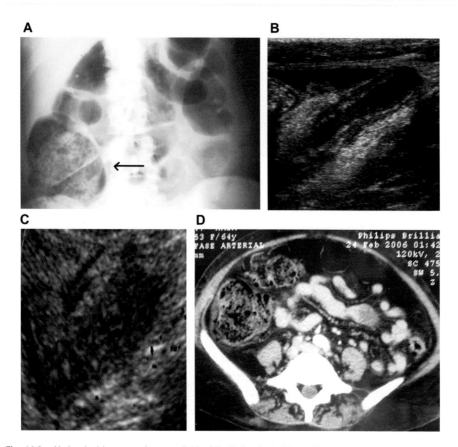

Fig. 14.6 Abdominal images of appendicitis. (A) Abdominal plain radiography showing distension of the cecum with fecal loading image. (B) Abdominal ultrasound showing an enlarged appendix with a thick wall. (C) Doppler ultrasound showing an inflamed appendix. (D) Computed tomography of a patient with appendicitis. Observe the fecal loading in the cecum. (From Petroianu A. Diagnosis of acute appendicitis. *Int J Surg.* 2012;10(3):115–119 [Fig. 2]. ISSN 1743-9191, https://doi.org/10.1016/j.ijsu.2012.02.006, http://www.sciencedirect.com/science/article/pii/S1743919112000246.)

against exploratory laparotomy/laparoscopy (e.g., anticoagulation, recent myocardial infarction) (Fig. 14.8).

DIFFERENTIAL DIAGNOSIS

Most causes of acute abdominal pain can mimic acute appendicitis. Most commonly, acute gastroenteritis, inflammatory bowel disease, right-sided diverticulitis, irritable bowel syndrome, ectopic pregnancy, ischemic colitis, psoas abscess, and mesenteric artery ischemia are misdiagnosed as diverticulitis. Black widow spider envenomation has also been misdiagnosed as acute appendicitis.

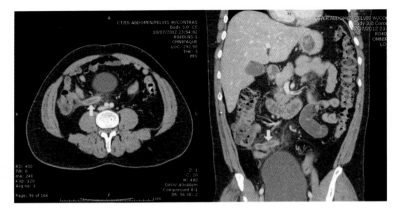

Fig. 14.7 Computed tomography (CT) scan images (axial (left image) and coronal sections (right image)) demonstrating a dilated appendix, with adjacent fat stranding, suggestive of mild acute appendicitis. *Arrows*, Dilated appendix. (From Teixeira PGR. Demetrios demetriades, appendicitis: changing perspectives. *Adv Surg.* 2013;47(1):119–140.)

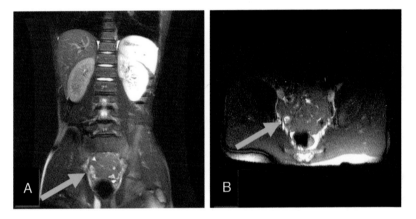

Fig. 14.8 (A) Magnetic resonance imaging (MRI) abdomen demonstrating acute, nonperforated appendicitis. MRI of abdomen of an 11-year-old boy with a 14-hour history of right lower quadrant abdominal pain. (B) MRI demonstrated an 8-mm appendix with periappendiceal fluid. (From Murphy EEK, Berman L. Clinical evaluation of acute appendicitis. *Clin Pediatr Emerg Med.* 2014;15(3):223–230.)

Because the pain of acute herpes zoster may precede the rash by 3 to 5 days, it may erroneously be attributed to acute appendicitis.

TREATMENT

Any discussion regarding the treatment of acute appendicitis is that appendectomy remains the only 100% curative treatment (Fig. 14.9). That being said,

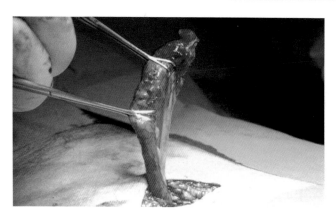

Fig. 14.9 Acute appendicitis as seen at surgery. (From Sugrue C, Hogan A, Robertson I, et al. Incisional hernia appendicitis: a report of two unique cases and literature review. *Int J Surg Case Rep.* 2013;4(3):256–258.)

recent experience suggests that many treatment decisions regarding patients suffering from acute appendicitis are based on traditions, many of which find their origins in the preantibiotic era, rather than evidence-based medicine. These traditions are reinforced by the belief held by both the lay public and medical professionals that appendectomy is a benign procedure. Current clinical thinking suggests that the best outcomes for patients with acute appendicitis can be obtained by subsetting the individual patient into one of three groups: (1) patients with mild acute appendicitis with a small phlegmon or abscess, (2) patients with more severe acute appendicitis with a well-defined abscess that is anatomically amenable to percutaneous draining, and (3) patients with severe systemic symptoms and larger multicompartmental or multiple abscesses not amenable to percutaneous drainage (Figs. 14.10 and 14.11; see also Fig. 14.9). This subsetting allows a more rational timing of appendectomy that has the potential to significantly reduce the mortality and morbidity associated with both the disease and the surgery. Patients in all groups are treated with antibiotics that cover both aerobic and anaerobic microbes. Patients in group 1 are allowed to recover from their acute illness, and an interval appendectomy can be performed under ideal anesthetic and operative conditions (e.g., empty stomach, normal hydration, blood sugar control, discontinuation of anticoagulants, and antiplatelet medications). Group 2 can be treated with emergent percutaneous drainage of a well-defined abscess, and interval appendectomy can be performed after fistula closure. Group 3 requires urgent surgical intervention in all circumstances. It should be noted that there are some additional advantages to appendectomy, including the opportunity for the surgeon to evaluate the entire abdomen at the time of surgery to correct the working diagnosis; to identify coexistent occult pathology; and to remove appendiceal tissue containing

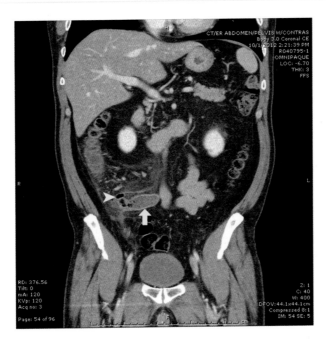

Fig. 14.10 Computed tomography (CT) scan: coronal section image demonstrating a dilated appendix with periappendicular fat stranding and extraluminal gas suggestive of perforated appendicitis. *Arrow*, Dilated appendix; *arrowhead*, extraluminal gas. (From Teixeira PGR. Demetrios demetriades, appendicitis: changing perspectives. *Adv Surg.* 2013;47(1):119–140.)

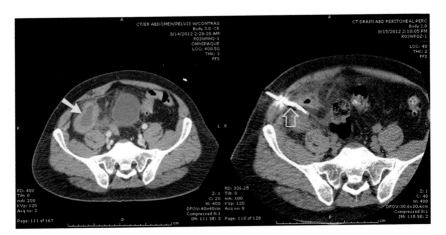

Fig. 14.11 Computed tomography (CT) scan axial images demonstrating perforated appendicitis with abscess *(left)* and percutaneous CT-guided drainage of the abscess *(right)*. *Arrow*, Abscess; *empty arrow*, percutaneous catheter insertion. (From Teixeira PGR. Demetrios demetriades, appendicitis: changing perspectives. *Adv Surg.* 2013;47(1):119–140.)

malignant cells (e.g., adenocarcinoma and carcinoid, which have an incidence of 0.7% and 0.07%, respectively).

HIGH-YIELD TAKEAWAYS

- The patient is febrile.
- The patient's symptomatology is consistent with acute appendicitis.
- The patient's physical exam is consistent with acute appendicitis.
- CT scanning of the abdomen is the preferred imaging modality to diagnose acute appendicitis with an accuracy of 98%, although ultrasound imaging is also useful and avoids radiation exposure for the patient.
- Physical diagnosis is useful in the diagnosis of appendix pain.

Suggested Readings

Al-Faouri AF, Ajarma KY, Al-Abbadi AM, et al. The Alvarado score versus computed tomography in the diagnosis of acute appendicitis: a prospective study. *Med J Armed Forces India*. 2016;72(4):332–337.

Debnath J, Sharma V, Ravikumar R, et al. Clinical mimics of acute appendicitis: is there any role of imaging? *Med J Armed Forces India*. 2016;72(3):285–292.

Lourenco P, Brown J, Leipsic J, et al. The current utility of ultrasound in the diagnosis of acute appendicitis. *Clin Imaging*. 2016;40(5):944–948.

Pisano M, Capponi MG, Ansaloni L. Acute appendicitis: an open issue. Current trends in diagnostic and therapeutic options. In: Kon K, Rai M, eds. *Microbiology for Surgical Infections*. Amsterdam: Academic Press; 2014:97–110.

Romero J, Valencia S, Guerrero A. Acute appendicitis during coronavirus disease 2019 (COVID-19): changes in clinical presentation and CT findings. *J Am Coll Radiol*. 2020;17(8):1011–1013.

Waldman SD. Acute appendicitis. In: *Atlas of Common Pain Syndromes*. ed. 4. Philadelphia: Elsevier; 2019:306–310.

Mai Huang

A 64-Year-Old Waitress With Left-Sided Abdominal Pain and Fever

- Learn the common causes of abdominal pain.
- Develop an understanding of the unique anatomy of the colon.
- Develop an understanding of the causes of diverticulitis.
- Develop an understanding of the differential diagnosis of diverticulitis.
- Learn the clinical presentation of diverticulitis.
- Learn how to examine the abdomen.
- Learn how to use physical examination to identify diverticulitis.
- Develop an understanding of the treatment options for diverticulitis.

Mai Huang

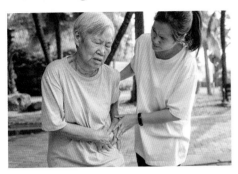 Mai Huang is a 64-year-old waitress with the chief complaint of, "My belly hurts." Mai stated that over the past week or so, she felt constipated, and for the last few days, she's been experiencing crampy pain in her left lower abdomen. Mai stated that she woke up today feeling like she had the stomach flu and felt like she had a fever. She called her daughter, who said that Mai probably had appendicitis and that she needed to go to the emergency room. Instead she called our office, and we worked her in. "Doctor, I am so sorry to bother you. I am sure this is nothing. I just wanted to be able to tell my daughter Sally that it was just the flu. You know how daughters can be." I reassured her that I understood and would do everything I could to get things sorted out, and if she wanted I'd be happy to give Sally a call. "So, Mai, have you ever had anything like this before?" She said, "No Doctor, never." I asked, "Have you had any previous abdominal pain?" She replied, "No, never."

I asked Mai what made the pain worse, and she said that when she came over to the office on the bus, every time the bus hit a bump, it would jar her belly and make it hurt. "Also, Doctor, and this is embarrassing, I am having a lot of gas." I asked, "Anything else?" She said that she felt like she was bloated, but really any activity made the pain worse. I asked her what made the pain better, and she said that she tried to drink some hot tea because she didn't have much of an appetite, but the pain just wasn't getting any better. In fact, it seemed to be a little worse. Mai denied significant sleep disturbance.

I asked Mai to point with one finger to show me where it hurt the most, and she immediately pointed to her left lower quadrant.

On physical examination, Mai was febrile, with a temperature of 100.6°F. Her respirations were 18, and her pulse was 78 and regular. Her blood pressure was 106/72. Mai's head, eyes, ears, nose, throat (HEENT) exam was normal, as was her cardiopulmonary examination. Her thyroid was normal. Her abdominal examination revealed tenderness in the left lower quadrant, and I thought that I could feel a mass. Bowel sounds were diminished, with no organomegaly. Mai had mild costovertebral angle (CVA) tenderness on the left. There was no peripheral edema. Her low back examination was normal. Visual inspection of the abdomen was unremarkable. A careful neurologic examination was normal.

Key Clinical Points—What's Important and What's Not
THE HISTORY

- Several-day history of change in bowel habits, with constipation and later increased flatulence
- Fever
- Left-sided abdominal pain that is worsening
- Feeling systemically ill
- Pain made worse by activity or doing things that jar the abdomen
- No other past history of abdominal pain

THE PHYSICAL EXAMINATION

- Patient is febrile
- Obvious tenderness in the left lower quadrant
- Palpation of a mass in the left lower quadrant
- Hypoactive bowel sounds
- Left CVA tenderness

OHER FINDINGS OF NOTE

- Normal HEENT examination
- Normal cardiovascular examination
- Normal pulmonary examination
- No peripheral edema
- Normal neurologic examination

 ## What Tests Would You Like to Order?

The following tests were ordered:
- Computed tomography (CT) of the abdomen

TEST RESULTS

CT scanning with contrast enhancement revealed perforated diverticulitis of the sigmoid as evidenced by extraluminal gas and fluid surrounding the sigmoid colon, as well as the finding of extraluminal fecal bowel contents near the site of perforation (Fig. 15.1).

 ## Clinical Correlation—Putting It All Together

What is the diagnosis?
- Diverticulitis with perforation

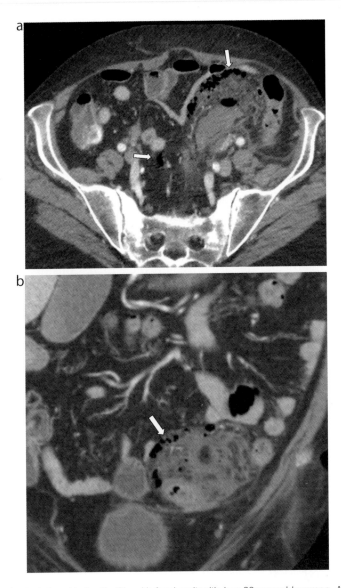

Fig. 15.1 Perforated sigmoid diverticulitis with fecal peritonitis in a 60-year-old woman. Axial contrast-enhanced computed tomography (CECT) shows loculated extraluminal gas and fluid surrounding the sigmoid colon and in the central pelvis (*arrows*, a). Coronal CECT image shows extraluminal bowel contents (*arrow*, b) near the site of perforation. A 2-cm colotomy in the sigmoid colon actively leaking fecal material was seen at surgery, at which time a sigmoid colectomy was performed. (From Sugi MD, Sun DC, Menias CO, et al. Acute diverticulitis: key features for guiding clinical management. *Eur J Radiol.* 2020;128:109026 [Fig. 6]. ISSN 0720-048X, https://doi.org/10.1016/j.ejrad.2020.109026, http://www.sciencedirect.com/science/article/pii/S0720048X20302151.)

The Science Behind the Diagnosis

CLINICAL SYNDROME

Diverticulitis is a common cause of acute abdominal pain in Western and industrialized countries. Found more commonly in women, the disease occurs more commonly after the fourth decade. Diverticulitis occurs when small herniations of the colonic mucosa and submucosa, known as diverticula, become inflamed or tear (Fig. 15.2). It is estimated that approximately 75% of patients will have diverticula by the age of 80, as there is age-related weakening of the abdominal wall in areas of insertion of the vasa recta. Decreased bowel motility of senescence may also play a role in increasing intracolonic pressure, as may changes in the microbiome of the gastrointestinal tract.

Patients with diverticulitis will develop abdominal pain that is usually located in the left lower quadrant, although there is an increased incidence of right-sided diverticular disease in Asians (Fig. 15.3). Constipation is present approximately 50% of the time, with diarrhea occurring in 25% of patients suffering from acute diverticulitis. Abdominal tenderness is invariably present, as are fever and chills. The pain of diverticulitis is proportional to the extent of inflammation, with the pain ranging from mild, intermittent pain to severe, unremitting pain with frank signs of peritonitis, including rebound tenderness. Lower gastrointestinal bleed, which may be significant, may also be present.

Factors that increase the risk of developing diverticulitis include advancing age, low-fiber/high-fat diet, obesity, smoking, and the use of corticosteroids and nonsteroidal antiinflammatory agents. Diets high in vitamin D and the use of statins and calcium channel blockers may exert a protective effect. Mild cases of diverticulitis are managed conservatively, but approximately 25% of patients with acute diverticulitis will develop complications that may include abscess formation, bowel obstruction, peritonitis, and sepsis.

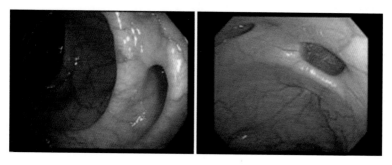

Fig. 15.2 Diverticulosis on colonoscopy. (From Feuerstein JD, Falchuk KR. Diverticulosis and diverticulitis. *Mayo Clin Proc.* 2016;91(8):1094−1104.)

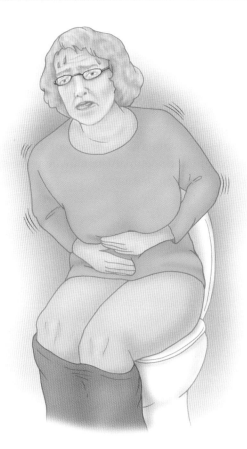

Fig. 15.3   The patient with acute diverticulitis will suffer from left-sided abdominal pain associated with a change in bowel habits. Fever and chills are often present. (From Waldman S. *Atlas of Common Pain Syndromes*. ed. 4. Philadelphia: Elsevier; 2019 [Fig. 78-2].)

SIGNS AND SYMPTOMS

Left-sided abdominal pain is present in most patients with acute diverticulitis, although patients of Asian descent have an increased incidence of right-sided diverticulitis, which may mimic acute appendicitis. The pain of acute diverticulitis is associated with anorexia and a change in bowel habits and gastrointestinal symptoms of constipation, diarrhea, bloating, flatulence, and nausea and vomiting. A small percentage of patients will complain of urinary urgency and frequency secondary to irritation of the adjacent urinary tract. Often, the patient will flex the hip on the affected side owing to irritation of the psoas muscle. Mild diverticulitis may produce minimal constitutional symptoms, but if the disease progresses, fever and chills may be pronounced.

On physical examination, the extent of abdominal findings will be in proportion to the extent of the diverticulitis. Small microperforations of left-sided diverticula will produce diffuse left lower quadrant pain with minimal peritoneal findings. With more severe diverticulitis, the pain will become more localized to the left lower quadrant and pelvis, with rebound tenderness and prominent physical findings. If a peridiverticular abscess or phlegmon forms, a tender, palpable mass may be identified. The abdomen may be distended and tympanic to percussion, with bowel sounds diminished or absent. If a fistula into the genitourinary tract forms, fecaluria or pneumaturia may be present, with colovaginal fistulas occurring in females (Figs. 15.4 and 15.5).

TESTING

CT of the abdomen and pelvis has replaced barium enema as the preferred imaging modality to diagnose diverticulitis because not only can it diagnose the disease with a high degree of specificity and sensitivity, but it can also identify complications as well as pericolonic abscess and other pathologic processes that may mimic diverticulitis. The Hinchey classification can help define the severity of complicated diverticulitis and guide treatment (Box 15.1 and Fig. 15.6). Ultrasonography and colonoscopy can also diagnose diverticulitis but cannot identify such potential serious complications as intraabdominal or retroperitoneal abscess or fecal peritonitis (Fig. 15.7). Based on the patient's clinical presentation, additional testing (complete blood count to identify leukocytosis with a left shift, urinalysis, and serum chemistries) is indicated. Blood cultures should be obtained if fever is present. A pregnancy test must be obtained on all females of child bearing age to rule out ectopic pregnancy. If abscess formation is suspected, imaging of adjacent structures (e.g., hip, bladder) should be obtained sooner rather than later.

DIFFERENTIAL DIAGNOSIS

Many causes of acute abdominal pain can mimic diverticulitis (Box 15.2). Most commonly, acute gastroenteritis, inflammatory bowel disease, irritable bowel syndrome, ectopic pregnancy, ischemic colitis, and mesenteric artery ischemia are misdiagnosed as diverticulitis. Acute appendicitis can also mimic right-sided diverticulitis.

TREATMENT

The treatment of diverticulitis is based on the severity of the disease and must be individualized to the specific patient. In uncomplicated diverticulitis presenting with mild symptoms, patients are treated with a clear liquid diet for 7 to 10 days

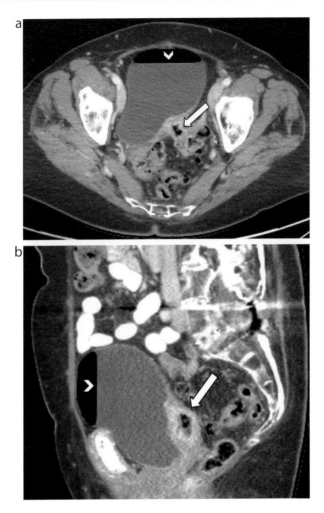

Fig. 15.4 Colovesical fistula due to sigmoid diverticulitis. (a) Axial and sagittal (b) contrast-enhanced computed tomography images show a mural abscess and thick-walled fistulous tract between the sigmoid colon and urinary bladder (*arrows*, a-b) and an air-fluid level in the bladder (*arrowheads*, a-b). (From Sugi MD, Sun DC, Menias CO, et al. Acute diverticulitis: key features for guiding clinical management. *Eur J Radiol.* 2020;128:109026 [Fig. 10]. ISSN 0720-048X, https://doi.org/10.1016/j.ejrad.2020.109026, http://www.sciencedirect.com/science/article/pii/S0720048X20302151.)

and oral broad-spectrum antibiotics, such as ciprofloxacin and metronidazole, that cover anaerobic microorganisms. Opioids should be avoided, as they decrease bowel motility.

For patients with more severe symptomatology, including fever and chills, the immediate use of broad-spectrum intravenous antibiotics and the drainage of any abscess are mandatory (Fig. 15.8). If the abscess cannot be drained

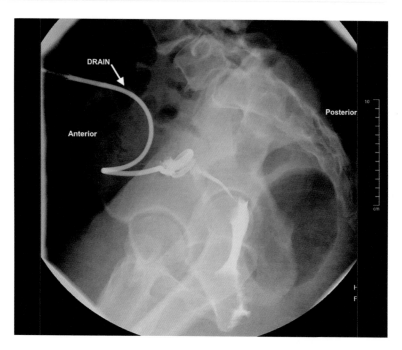

Fig. 15.5 Sagittal view of sinogram through a percutaneous drain demonstrated connection between the diverticular abscess and vagina. (From Rook JM, Dworsky JQ, Curran T, et al. Elective surgical management of diverticulitis. *Curr Prob Surg.* 2020:100876 [Fig. 4]. ISSN 0011-3840, https://doi.org/10.1016/j.cpsurg.2020.100876, http://www.sciencedirect.com/science/article/pii/S0011384020301465.)

BOX 15.1 ■ Hinchley Classification of Diverticulitis	
Stage I	Pericolic abscess or phlegmon
Stage II	Pelvic, intraabdominal, or retroperitoneal abscess
Stage III	Generalized purulent peritonitis
Stage IV	Generalized fecal peritonitis

percutaneously, or if significant perforation, fistula, or bowel obstruction is present, emergent surgical treatment consisting of primary bowel resection is indicated (Fig. 15.9). Occasionally, a diverting colostomy will be required to allow resolution of severe diverticulitis (Fig. 15.10).

COMPLICATIONS AND PITFALLS

Diverticulitis is a common cause of acute abdominal pain. Its clinical presentation can range from a mild self-limited disease to a life-threatening illness. Because of

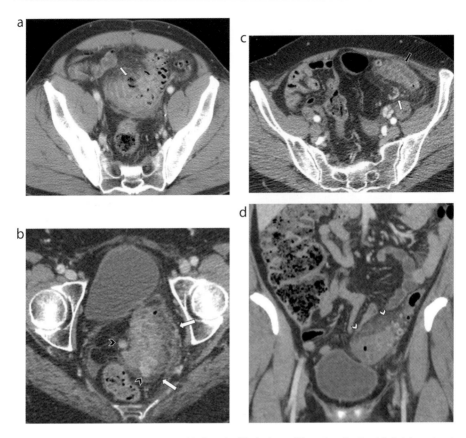

Fig. 15.6 Acute uncomplicated sigmoid diverticulitis in four different patients. (a) Axial contrast-enhanced computed tomography (CECT) image shows wall thickening of the sigmoid colon and fat stranding centered around a diverticulum *(arrow)* in a 65-year-old man. (b) Axial CECT shows inflammatory pericolic fat stranding *(arrows)* around the sigmoid colon with several hyperdense diverticula *(arrowheads)* in a 76-year-old woman. (c) Axial CECT shows engorgement of the mesenteric veins *(white arrow)* draining a mildly inflamed segment of sigmoid colon *(black arrow)* in a 57-year-old man. (d) Coronal CECT shows multiple diverticula arising from the sigmoid colon, which is mildly thickened, with confluent inflammatory stranding of the pericolic fat *(arrowheads)* in a 37-year-old woman. (From Sugi MD, Sun DC, Menias CO, et al. Acute diverticulitis: key features for guiding clinical management. *Eur J Radiol.* 2020;128:109026 [Fig. 3]. ISSN 0720-048X, https://doi.org/10.1016/j.ejrad.2020.109026, http://www.sciencedirect.com/science/article/pii/S0720048X20302151.)

the number of other diseases that mimic diverticulitis, diagnosis and treatment may be delayed, leading to increased morbidity and rarely, mortality. Early implementation of broad-spectrum antibiotics and identification and drainage of pericolonic abscess are mandatory to decrease more severe complications.

Many other causes of an acute abdomen can mimic the presentation of diverticulitis. The failure to correctly identify the source of the patient's abdominal

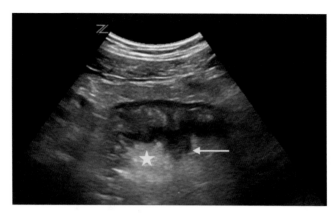

Fig. 15.7 Diverticulitis on ultrasonography. The arrow indicates a diverticulum with associated bowel wall edema. The star indicates pericolonic infiltration observed as hyperechoic fat. (From Cohen A, Li T, Stankard B, et al. A prospective evaluation of point-of-care ultrasonographic diagnosis of diverticulitis in the emergency department. *Ann Emerg Med*. 2020 [Fig. 1]. ISSN 0196-0644, https://doi.org/10.1016/j.annemergmed.2020.05.017, http://www.sciencedirect.com/science/article/pii/S0196064420303656.)

BOX 15.2 ■ Diseases That May Mimic Acute Diverticulitis

Appendicitis
Inflammatory bowel disease
Irritable bowel syndrome
Colorectal malignancies
Acute gastroenteritis
Ectopic pregnancy
Ischemic colitis
Abdominal angina
Tuboovarian abscess
Pelvic inflammatory disease
Ureteral calculi
Volvulus
Ovarian torsion
Endometriosis

---

symptoms can lead to significant morbidity and mortality. It should be remembered that right-sided diverticulitis is common in patients of Asian descent and may present identically to acute appendicitis. Early identification and drainage of abscess is essential to avoid more serious complications when treating diverticulitis.

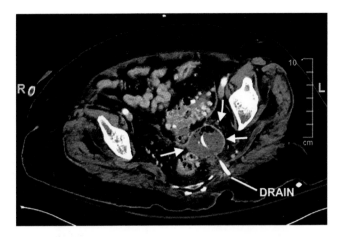

Fig. 15.8 Computed tomography of the pelvis demonstrates a transgluteal percutaneous drain within a diverticular pelvic abscess *(arrows)*. (From Rook JM, Dworsky JQ, Curran T, et al. Elective surgical management of diverticulitis. *Curr Prob Surg*. 2020:100876 [Fig. 2]. ISSN 0011-3840, https://doi.org/10.1016/j.cpsurg.2020.100876, http://www.sciencedirect.com/science/article/pii/S0011384020301465.)

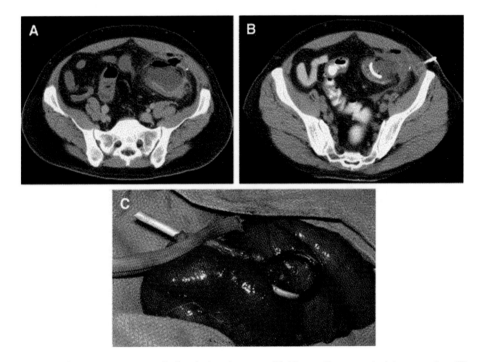

Fig. 15.9 Surgical treatment of diverticular abscess. (A) Diagnostic computed tomography. (B) Percutaneous drain placed. (C) Intraoperative resection of bowel with percutaneous drain in place. (From Chapman JR, Wolff BG. The management of complicated diverticulitis. *Adv Surg*. 2006;40:285−297.)

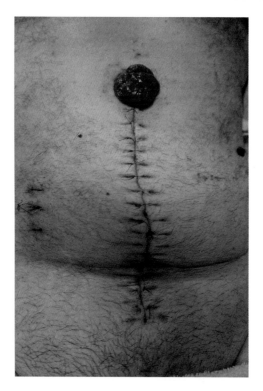

Fig. 15.10 Diverting transverse colostomy. (From Sugarbaker PH. Diverting transverse colostomy in a midline incision, a case report. *Int J Surg Open*. 2019;16:14-17 [Fig. 2]. ISSN 2405-8572, https://doi.org/10.1016/j.ijso.2018.11.007, http://www.sciencedirect.com/science/article/pii/S2405857218300998.)

HIGH-YIELD TAKEAWAYS

- The patient is febrile, which is always a concern in a patient with abdominal pain.
- The patient's symptomatology is most consistent with acute diverticulitis, and physical examination and testing should focus on the confirmation of this working diagnosis and to rule out other diseases that may mimic the clinical presentation of diverticulitis.
- The patient has left lower quadrant tenderness, which is highly suggestive of diverticulitis.
- There is a mass in the left lower quadrant, which in this clinical setting is most likely an abscess.

(*Continued*)

- CT scanning will provide high-yield information regarding the source of the patient's signs and symptoms and is highly accurate in confirming the diagnosis of diverticulitis, as well as identifying associated complications such as abscess and fistula formation.

Suggested Readings

Curran T, Kwaan MR. Controversies in the management of diverticulitis. *Adv Surg.* 2020;54:1–16.

Ferrara F, Bollo J, Vanni LV, et al. Diagnosis and management of right colonic diverticular disease: a review. *Cir Esp.* 2016;94(10):553–559.

Feuerstein JD, Falchuk KR. Diverticulosis and diverticulitis. *Mayo Clin Proc.* 2016;91 (8):1094–1104.

Horesh N, Wasserberg N, Zbar AP, et al. Changing paradigms in the management of diverticulitis. *Int J Surg.* 2016;33(Pt A):146–150.

Peery AF, Keku TO, Martin CF, et al. Distribution and characteristics of colonic diverticula in a United States screening population. *Clin Gastroenterol Hepatol.* 2016;14 (7):980–985.

Roig JV, Salvador A, Frasson M, et al. Surgical treatment of acute diverticulitis. A retrospective multicentre study. *Cir Esp.* 2016;94(10):569–577.

Tan JPL, Barazanchi AWH, Singh PP, et al. Predictors of acute diverticulitis severity: a systematic review. *Int J Surg.* 2016;26:43–52.

Note: Page numbers followed by '*f*' indicate figures; those followed by '*t*' indicate tables and '*b*' indicate boxes.